You Care *Too* Much

CREATIVE WOMEN ON
THE QUESTION OF SELF CARE

PUBLISHED BY

**with/out
pret/end**

6   PERSONAL ESSAY
CARE / CARRY / CURE   Jessika Hepburn
How do I choose what to care for? How much can I possibly carry?

16   POETRY
MIKVAH   Leah Horlick
The hole in the floor is in my body. My body, the reminder we will someday crawl out.

24   PERSONAL ESSAY
THESE DAYS   Anabela Piersol
I needed to feel safe from conversations and images that cropped up like landmines.

32   PHOTOGRAPHY
THE STUFF THAT FEEDS US
Vicky Lam, Jen Spinner and Christina Yan
Finding the balance between on-the-go and stay-for-cake.

38   ART
PAPER CUTS   Winnie Truong
Creating new shapes that challenge status quo ideas of beauty and discomfort.

46   FICTION
FALL IN LOVE IF YOU'RE SO UNHAPPY   Sofia Mostaghimi
We met unromantically by swiping right instead of left on each other's profile pictures.

58   PERSONAL ESSAY
MY LEFT FIST   Naomi Moyer
The emotional adversity, my depression — they were stuck between my fingers and my palm.

66   POETRY
IF DEATH THEN LOVE | IF THIRTY THEN THIRTY-ONE   Brooke Manning
You spend weeks, months, years, questioning the reality of the event.

PERSONAL ESSAY
74 #SOFTASFUCK Nada Alic
Softness can exist in your favorite record or linen sheets or inside a delicious sandwich.

PHOTO ESSAY
80 WEEKENDS Angela Lewis
Love and obligation: An intimate story of a daughter caring for her mother.

ILLUSTRATION
88 SELF CARE AND HEALTH Tallulah Fontaine
Slowing down long enough to notice the things that bring peace.

FLORAL SCULPTURE
92 HOW CAN YOU SAY NO TO THAT? Kathryn Bondy
Embracing the recurring cycles of growth and decay.

FICTION
96 BECOMING CARYS Erin Klassen
I used to think that we were born with maps inside us, telling us who to become.

PERSONAL ESSAY
110 MY GRANDFATHER'S HOUSE Adina Tarralik Duffy
You are as far away as the moon and as close to your roots as if sleeping in your mother's womb.

PERSONAL ESSAY
118 THE PLACE WE MET Mo Handahu
This is where we felt vulnerable but safe. Not our best, but getting better.

Front cover and photo series, *It's Only Natural*, throughout: by Angela Lewis.
Back cover photo: by Vicky Lam; styling by Christina Yan.

"Your hand opens and closes, opens and closes. If it were always a fist or always stretched open, you would be paralysed. Your deepest presence is in every small contracting and expanding, the two as beautifully balanced and coordinated as birds' wings." —*Rumi*

"Who cares?" I've never understood that apathetic proclamation, oft grunted by the series of Nirvana fans I dated in highschool. Maybe that's because I've always cared, so much, about everything.

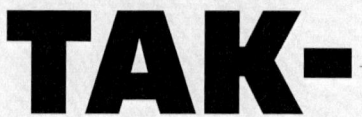

By everything, I mean: He didn't call, I'm running late, I can't believe that Ross and Rachel broke up, the recipe calls for crème fraîche — don't you *dare* use ricotta. I care about important things, too: A friend is feeling down, I should call my brother more often, global warming is real, gun violence continues to terrorize.

I learned to be this way from watching my mother who is an expert at caring too much. Growing up, I saw her scrub the house when company was coming, pack us bagged lunches every morning before school, silently curse her reflection in the mirror while dressing for one of my father's corporate functions, hem and haw over which colour to paint the front foyer. She was the best soprano in the church choir; she hosted out-of-town family for the holidays; she memorized everyone's phone number and birthdate and least favourite foods, she held me close when I cried.

My mother was and is, in my experience, the most generous, caring person on the planet. She knew what everyone around her needed to feel comfortable, happy, safe and challenged — and yet, I never once saw her apply this caliber of care to herself. And the consequences were tragic. By my mid-teens she had reached her capacity for giving herself away, as she had done for everyone in her world for so many years, without speaking up to ask for the things she needed to feel whole. Drinking seemed like the only option that could offer a temporary escape to her internal prison — that is until it almost killed her.

Mom is doing great now, but she had to learn the importance of self care the hard way, and by watching her, I did too. Self-care™ has since become a buzzword — Listicles, Instagram, and Gwyneth Paltrow tell us to take a minute, have a bath, get a pedicure — we deserve it. But where is the guide that will lead us to real healing, when we're faced with the moments we need it most?

My tendency to care too much — about what people think, what they want, and who I should be still holds court more often than I'd like. At the same time, having empathy for others helps me develop wisdom — about myself and the communities I belong to. In this book, contributors consider how their approach to self care takes shape in the 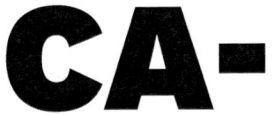 face of loss, mental illness, trauma and while struggling to find the balance between too much and not enough. Future generations will have to care about the big issues facing our world. The caring we do, for each other and ourselves, needs to exist in balance. We'll need to learn to turn inward, to listen to the voices within telling us how to be our best selves. And we'll need to be ready for the answers. —**ERIN KLASSEN** *editor*

Working with Erin on this anthology has been gratifying in ways I almost forgot existed — I've been doing what I do for a long time. That is, making imagery and creating layouts in the sometimes strict boundaries of commercial art. Being given the freedom and trust by an editor to try new things and get uncomfortable reminds me of why I started creating imagery in the first place. It's truly exhilarating to make media designed to evoke deep emotions in readers.

Erin and I loved the idea of commissioning photography to visually introduce each written piece. For us, it was an obvious choice to engage photographer Angela Lewis who was already contributing to the book. Her ability to tease out whimsical moments with her subjects is unique and admirable. Between the three of us, we decided to depict nude models in nature, using a graphic style that would lend itself well to our black and 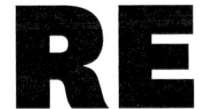 white format. We felt that a natural setting was ideal to explore issues of self care. Being naked in the outdoors is both freeing and scary! In both a literal and symbolic sense — there's nowhere to hide except within yourself. The pieces came together: A private location in the country, two beautifully strong women to pose for us and perfect weather on the day of the shoot. Angela created *It's Only Natural*, a stunning and mysterious series of portraits that brush against you with a hint of the words to come.

As a team, we consciously engaged a woman of colour and a Caucasian woman to be our models. When settling on the final photo selections, I was achingly aware that we would need to consider the range of cultural and racial diversity of our contributors. In some cases, it felt right to pair an image featuring our striking model of colour with a story by a woman of colour. For others, we chose the image that best represented the concepts rather than focusing so literally on race — an exposed neck, a protective curl, a playful dance. In all instances, we listened to our gut. I'm extremely proud of our collaboration and the safe space we created and maintained throughout the process. —**JEN SPINNER** *art director*

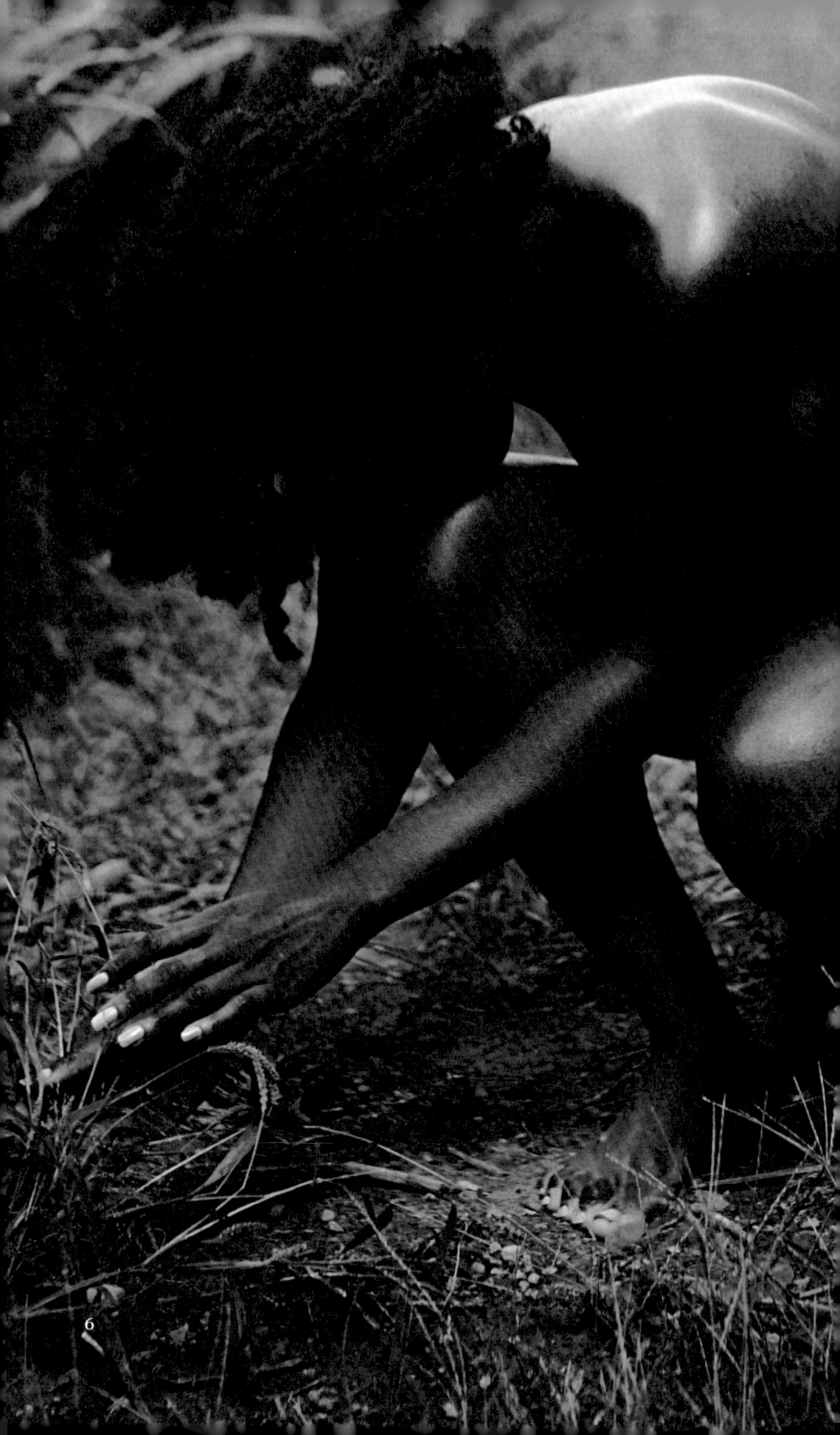

JESSIKA HEPBURN

thinks we could do better. That's why she's spent most of her life teaching others about the importance of inclusive community and building a culture of care. Jess is used to writing about social change but found it difficult to bare all about losing her partner's parents — the most stable family she's ever had. She describes the process of writing about herself as being naked in a room full of strangers who all have sticks, wondering — will they throw them at her, or make a fire to keep her warm? Jessika believes that our survival as a race is bound up in care for each other and she's composed this essay with courage and an open heart — a feat of personal activism.

Care / Carry / Cure
by Jessika Hepburn

CARE

One day Care (Cura) scooped up some mud from the bank of a river and sculpted a human being. While she was considering her creation Jupiter came along and Care asked him to bring the sculpture to life, he agreed quickly but when Care wanted to name the human after herself he disagreed. Terra, the life force of the earth emerged and joined the debate, since she gave her own body to create the human it should be named after her. Unable to resolve their conflict the deities asked Saturn to mediate and agreed to abide by his decision. Saturn ruled that since Jupiter had given his spirit to the human he would take back the soul after death, as Terra had given her body she would receive it back after death, but "Since Care first fashioned the human being, let her have and hold it as long as it lives."[1]

My love you are crying, finally, wrenchingly, shivering so hard I'm afraid you'll shatter into a million tiny pieces. We are lying in the spare bed at your parent's house with the August sun filtering through the window, the light luminous and sweet. I wrap my body around you tightly, trying to hold you together, press into the spaces between us and fill the broken places with care, as if I could protect us with the force of my love.

There is a small animal in your chest making pained sounds that escape through teeth clenched so tightly my jaw aches for you, if I could find the right key to the lock I would open the cage to your heart and hold it gently. The blue-green-grey curve of your eye is a watery ocean deep enough to drown in. I imagine myself a life raft, buoyant, keeping us afloat.

"I couldn't take care of them."

The words come out choked with the knowing that we can't save people no matter how much we love them. I want to suck that pain from you, pull the salty familiar grief into my own body, hold it inside the place I carried our daughters, take the raw ingredients of loss and spin the dark threads into myth. I want to sculpt us a new life from the shell of the old.

With your tears on my face I make promises to the memory of your parents, to take care of their boy, this family, our love, to have and to hold it as long as we live.

That night I curl myself around your back while you sleep and cry silently, the way women do when the weight of what they carry is too heavy for bearing.

CARRY

*What of the mother
whose house is in flames
and both of her children
are in their beds crying
and she loves them both
with the whole of her heart
but she knows she can only
carry one at a time?*[2]

My mother is outside on the back porch ugly crying with snot dripping down her face, on display for all the neighbours, killing our quiet night at home. I have just tucked my daughters into bed, I have done all of the things, I am weary beyond words and have nothing left to give. The person I want to be would be kind and say all the right things, but I am suddenly twelve years old and furious that it is never, even this one time, allowed to be about me.

This has been the hardest year of my life.

They say things, good or bad, come in threes but three deaths in three weeks seems overkill, more tragic movie than reality. Both my in-laws are dead in the same hospital, two weeks and one day apart. I made Chris stay home the week in-between so he was not on the job the day his co-worker fell off a ladder and died on impact. I touch wood and kiss the earth that he is safe, for now. It is too much, too quickly, but what choice is there? I want us to go to bed and wake up when it is all over, but I don't have the privilege or the luxury of not-caring. No warm bath or glass of wine is going to fix this. I endure and do what needs to be done. Death certificates, funeral arrangements, caterers for the double memorial service, the details of dying. Like Anne Sexton on burying her parents: "It is June. I am tired of being brave."

After each death I call my mother prepared for her tears and emotional need. Part of me is pragmatic about her capacity, but the little girl who wants to be taken care of is gullible and when she offers help I ask her to visit and hang out with the grandkids for a couple of weeks. Maybe this time it will be different...

It has been nine days.

The past explodes in me when I see my mother crying and the only thing that matters is making her stop. Now. Please for the love of all that is good, please stop making this harder.

I start screaming, she turns to poison, we know this dance.

> *Childhood abuse. Aunt Lizzy blowing her brains out in an LA bathtub. Rape. Nana starving herself to death. Love as immolation. His fists on my face. Drugs, both the doing and quitting of them. Sixteen and pregnant. The endless construction of myself as someone worth living for. Bearing my daughters. Carrying my mother. I am arrogant enough to think I can sculpt meaning from whatever dirt life throws me.*

Two and a half years ago the phone rang and a kind voice said *hurry*, and I did. Six hours driving through the January night to Prince Edward Island where my mother was on life support diagnosed with sepsis from an undetermined source. Was I the cause? Caring for my mother is a full-time occupation, a life sentence of indentured emotional labour. Earlier that year I had quit. According to the Internet, happiness requires 'removing toxic people' so I withdrew from the poison of our relationship to focus on my career and young family. Without care, my mother stopped caring for herself. Decades of celibacy got traded in for kinky strangers from online fetish sites. Eventually some asshole raped her and tore something inside. I had to hack into her email accounts and scroll through endless dick pics to find a reason for her sudden illness, stopping occasionally to throw up in the ICU bathroom.

That year I accepted responsibility for carrying the weight of my mother's life. I know the statistical outcomes for Black women living with mental illness. Daily I try to remind her why living is a good idea, practicing a steady patience pulled from some previously undiscovered reservoirs of strength. I log hundreds of hours on the phone listening to her complaints and concerns, trying to navigate PTSD, anxiety, and depression. When my mother-in-law started losing herself to dementia and father-in-law was diagnosed with lung disease I focused on my mom and the kids, leaving Chris to deal with his parents. On the bright June day his mother died we took our children to the hospital. They sat outside the room eating obscenely coloured popsicles while we viewed the body. Some images burn forever — you bending to kiss her forehead, our silence, the weight of it all.

We know this dance.

"Chris needs us." I am screaming: "Maybe he can teach you something about pain."

She is poison: "I know everything about pain. I watched my mother die then I had to deal with *you*."

I do not have compassion because I'm sixteen on the side of the highway where she left me between nowhere and nowhere PEI. Nowhere = now here, I can and do lose myself for years in the spaces between those words. My nana is dead. We are living with Keith, my twenty-seven-year-old junkie of a boyfriend who will start hitting me a few weeks later. I stick out my thumb and get a ride from the kindest woman who takes me to her house for the night where we drink tea and play drums with her little daughter. She teaches me to use a sandblaster and etch a mirror with a yin-yang on the centre. Balance for the chaos. Goodness for no good reason. Later that year Keith and I are living on Vancouver Island, as far from PEI as possible when he leaves me on the side of a highway too. Pregnant with blood in my mouth. The doctor points out the hairline fracture on the x-ray of my jaw,

I make up some story about how a kid on a swing kicked me and book an abortion as soon as possible.

I am too tired to play the apologetic daughter. Chris and I go to the beach that night and watch some kids set off fireworks in the dark. In the morning Chris drives my mother to get a bus back to the Island, she talks about herself the whole way there.

"Some things in life cannot be fixed. They can only be carried," writes Megan Devine.[3] But who lives and who dies? How do I choose what to care for? How much can I possibly carry? There is a terrible battle happening in my heart, the weight of choosing what to care about and who to show up for is heavy enough to crush my relentless optimism. I'm about ready to quit on my raw red heart, exhausted by the futility of loving people who will only die.

I lock the bathroom door and cry like a child. I am so tired. There is no one who can take care of me. My hands are too small and I will never be able to care for or carry it all at one time. It is June, I must be brave.

CURE

Is it my responsibility to brew compassion in my students? Is compassion a necessary entry into the world of service? Can compassion be crafted, nurtured? Or, is it the result of service, the aftermath of reaching out actively for another?[4]

I am watching my father-in-law breathe, a doctor who sacrificed himself to be of service, a good man who did his best and is still dying tragically. What good did caring do him? Is care a burden, a gift of service, or both? If there is a lesson or some grace in this I can't see it right now. Chris is taking our daughters to the memorial service for his mother and I am here at the hospital because it feels wrong to mourn the dead and leave his father alone when he is already leaving us. After forty-five years of marriage, his body, so incapable of processing her loss, is racing to catch up. As I watch the numbers flicker on the monitor it seems brutally cruel that hearts are so fragile, even the strongest ones stop eventually — an average human heart only gets 2.5 billion beats in a lifetime, which might seem like a lot, but when every day uses up 100,000 of them it adds up fast. We go along taking them for granted until suddenly, too late, we realize how precious and finite they are. Soon you and your sister will be holding his hands through the night, bracketing the bed like parentheses, containing a life. We will marvel at how his strong heart kept beating even after his broken lungs quit for good.

Everyone wants to be happy and carefree but are we willing to pay the price for it? I am thinking now of Goethe's Dr. Faustus who made a deal with the devil, giving up his soul to be freed from care. It took the death of an elderly couple and his own blindness to show Faust the price of carelessness. According to Goethe we have to wrestle the weight, the heavy anxious burden of caring, in order to convert it into a real concern for others. Not caring means we have killed the very thing that makes us human.

When we arrive at the hospital, a visitor is already there. She is the wife of a close friend and knows my father-in-law well enough to see obligation is the only force that will make him attend to his own care. Unpacking a tower of plastic containers, she describes exactly how the tenderloin was cooked, the steamed vegetables drenched in butter and soaked with love. He tastes everything and thanks her between bites. With the same practical tenderness she massages him gently as he sleeps later, caring for the caregiver.

"The dead don't need care," she says, and it is the truest thing I have ever heard. I hold the clean, bright taste of this truth in my mouth, rolling it around on my tongue like sacrament or salvation, words to keep the dark of indifference at bay.

We care and need care because we are alive. This sharp grief that comes in waves means I haven't yet executed the soft centre of my heart to avoid future pain. Both "care" and "cure" come from the same Ancient Roman roots, the Latin term "cura" that meant to be both afflicted with trouble or anxiety and devotion to the welfare of another. These two meanings seem in conflict unless care is the cure. I'm reminded of every small mercy life has provided, the gifts of presence and perfect timing, unexpected reminders of simple goodness that appear to save me from total despair with the awareness that we are here to love and be loved, to hold close what is good in each other while we can. Everything else is secondary.

I make good on my vows to the dead, taking Chris to the ocean and to bed at every opportunity, baptizing us with sweat and the sea. We stay up until dawn to watch the Perseids and make wishes on comet debris. At night I taste salt on my skin and promise again, again, again to have and to hold it as long as I live. ◐

---

[1] C.J. Hyginus & Hyginus, C. J. Myth of Care. 1976.
[2] Ani DiFranco, "School Night." 2001.
[3] Megan Devine, Refuge in Grief. 2016.
[4] Diana Feige, Be the Change: Teacher, Activist, Global Citizen. 2010.

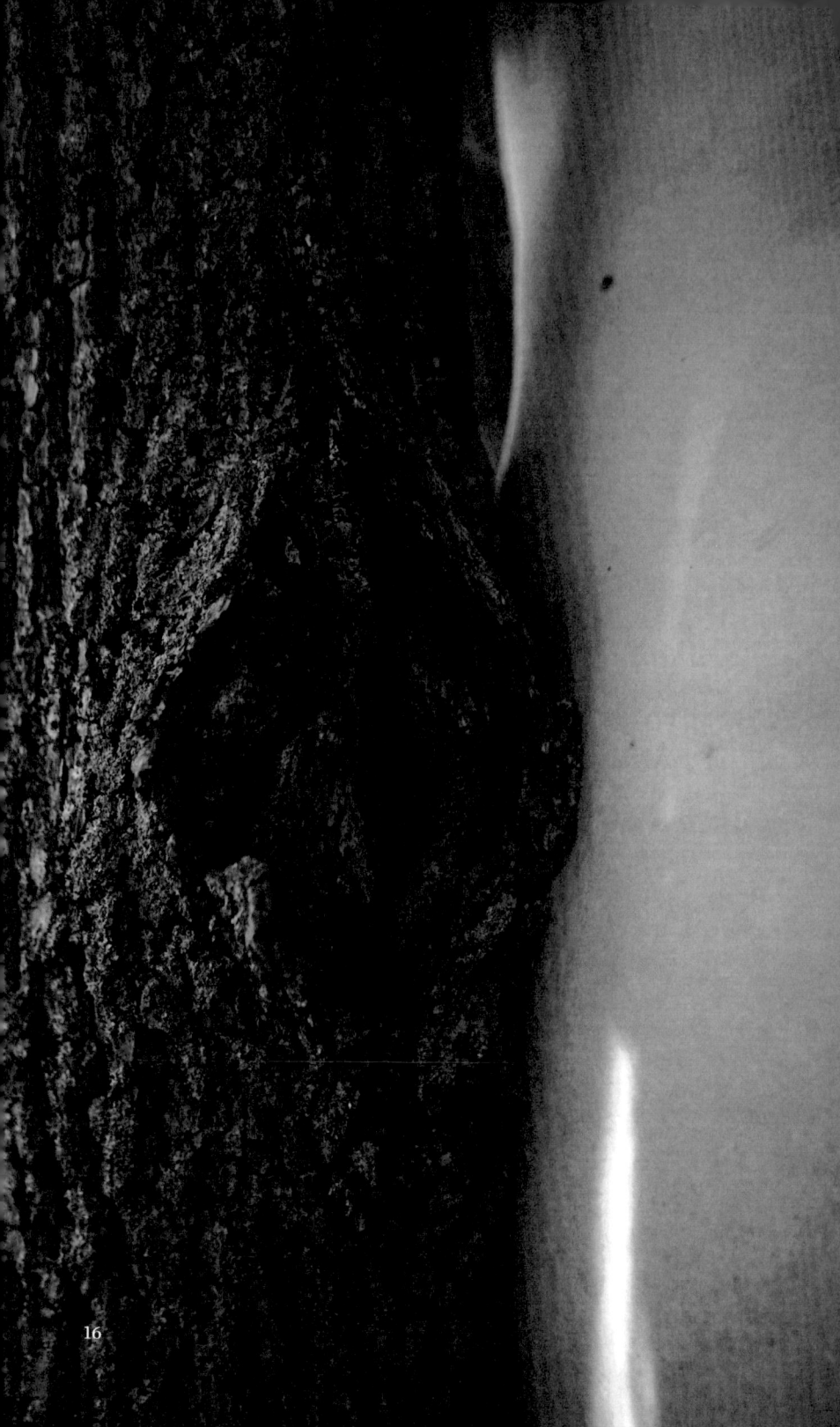

LEAH HORLICK

had her cards read in a scruffy East Van park by a queer witch who told her that her most recent book, *For Your Own Good,* was healing some old ancestral stuff in her family. Which made sense to the self-described Jewish femme, who sees her body as evidence of cultural survival. Leah is a lesbian poet who grew up in Saskatoon and is now living on the unceded Coast Salish territories in Vancouver. She believes that the trauma Jews have faced "gives us tremendous capacity to empathize with others." *Mikvah* looks at self care as legacy and proposes new approaches to healing. By looking back at the scripture that guided her ancestors, Leah shines a light on this important subject for future generations.

Mikvah

by Leah Horlick

"When I consider the work of your hands…"

I

It starts at the fence. The sky explosive
with light. I stand at the edge, beholding
chain link, its illusion of six corners. Shhh, helix.
I will not be sleeping here. I am so, so warm, the grass
alive with night and wet through my shoes. Look auntie.
I have shoes. As you close your eyes slowly in the chill of
death, at the edge of the fence, at the end of the war,
I am here at the freeway,
beneath the light. I stick the toe of my shoe in the fence.

Listen, there is only the shrieking of friends, and love, behind me.

II

The hole in the floor is in my body. The hole in the floor is old, old,
old country; it came from my grandmother's mouth. The hole
in the floor was for her great-grandmother, her sisters.
The hole in the floor is for women.

When the horses march up to the house, the hole
in the floor yawns wide. The hole
in the floor lives under the kitchen table,
gapes wide while the family eats, wider still when they starve.
Cold in the house, cold in the hole in the floor.
The hole in the floor is where the women go when
the Russians come.

The hole in the floor is where the women go. Hoofbeats. Cossacks.
Fur hats. A long tablecloth, white-knit lace draped to the floor,
hides the hole. If a black boot peeks under the lace. If a black glove
lifts the cloth. If a sharp woolen shoulder leans beneath the table
to inspect. A wooden floor, a perfectly hidden circle, or a dirt floor
with a carefully dirt-covered lid. The hole in the floor is why
I can't move. The hole in the floor is the bomb shelter. The hole in
the floor is the basement. The hole in the floor is wet with alcohol.
The hole in the floor is in my body. My body,
the reminder we will someday
crawl out.

III

In a crowd of people chanting, arms waving sharp angles,
fireworks, the roar, the heat, symmetry — a moment of possession.
Great-grandmother, it's you who has taught my body to escape.
To stand in this crowd, a shadow, quietly resisting even
the celebration of sameness by breathing, so ready to run.

IV

Where are you running to,
great-grandmother?
Grandchildren.

V

I eat. I eat. I eat. I never feel guilty
for eating.

"I slept but my heart was awake."

VI

We drive across the state of Florida, wet with heat, to visit
the cousin most revered in my childhood — her photos saintly
on the wall. *Hollywood*. The record still framed on her nursing
room wall. I hold the hand of the woman who held the hand of my
great-grandmother. This woman, my grandmother, my mother.
They sing an old, old song. It is impossible not to cry. Look.

VII

Look, great-zayde. Look, even as your daughter walks through
the valley of the Atlantic, even as you are bereaved by Catholicism,
look. Your grandchildren *are* Jewish, I promise. And like
golems I will carve a letter into the mud of your great-
grandchildren's foreheads.

VIII

But first, no more Philistines. No more words, drawn swords.
No more boys who think they speak Yiddish. No more mouths
who, when they kiss me, are only looking for oil.

IX

Let her kiss me with the kisses of her mouth.

X

Oh we are an old poem. The Black Sea, the Gulf.
Years of funeral fires and emperors, each mirage a regime.

Oh we are not the nuclear disaster they imagine. Your queen
was our queen and you are mine. It is so simple. Bread and fire,
olive and fig. Verses, pomegranate. Gold thread. The colour blue.

The sound *ch* at the beginning,
or the middle,
and the end of a word.

"This is my beloved, this is my friend."

XI
I am in love with the row of lights in your eyes. I am in love
with the muscle at the back of your neck, lioness. I am in love with
the flame at the end of the braid in your heart. I am in love with
your forearms, rods of gold set with topaz. I am in love with your
hands. Your mouth and the smoke that curls from it, the wine that
is the colour of your mouth. We are so, so old in love. When you
kiss me I can hear a millennia sing.

XII
The weight of our names in each hand. The right that is supposed
to be home, the left that is supposed to be home. At night we sit
and roll around difficult names in our mouths for our daughters
to be sure that each of our parents can pronounce them. I say
Tzipporah, you say *Zaporah*. I say, *loss*. You say, *this too shall pass*.

XIII
A miracle! Neither of us had been pregnant, neither did we know
the two children who came out of the room that had recently been
for the cat that morning. But we learned that they were yours
from their laugh — and because they were perfect.
How close they could grow to the fire without flinching,
the small golden scallops of wings on their chests.
How could this also be mine?

When they were afraid of the shower and didn't know why,
you said *Ask your mother*.

And when they came home from school one day and couldn't look
at the oven any more we both said *Not that kind of oven,
sweetheart*, and they touched my tattoos gently and you whispered
Not those, either. Every day we learn something so, so old through
their bodies. How could this, also, be mine?

XIV

How to explain to a child the inheritance
of this sound? My parents tell me it means
lily for years and years until I read —

Hebrew, weary; Akkadian, cow; Abyssinian, mistress.
Sold off in a fraudulent wedding, veiled from my sister's
lover, bartered by my father, eyes tender from crying
turned to varying ancient descriptions of blindness, visions.
The visions of a woman bearing child after child,
each one named for a wish.

May you be like her, they told me.
Why?

XV

So I'll come out the gate
knowing children are not the same
as love.

"If I forget you, Jerusalem."

XVI

Your labour camp is its own republic. The mass grave wants its independence. The Soviets still reaching that long, dead arm across the river. Abkhazia, Nagorno-Karabakh, South Ossetia. When you put your ear to the river you can hear footsteps walking around and around the Black Sea. Transnistria has its own president the same way Dachau is a town. Dachau was easier to visit. Children rode their tricycles around and around the camp. The nuns had taken a vow of silence, trying to reclaim something, their long habits sweeping the ruined ground.

XVII

Will we ever look at a fence, a shower
the same way? Tonight, the sky is explosive
with light.

XVIII

I take a handful of salt and throw it
gently down into that mouth of fear. We are women
who will not go back into the dirt that way. I will be
another kind of dust,
I promise.

XIX

We crawl out.

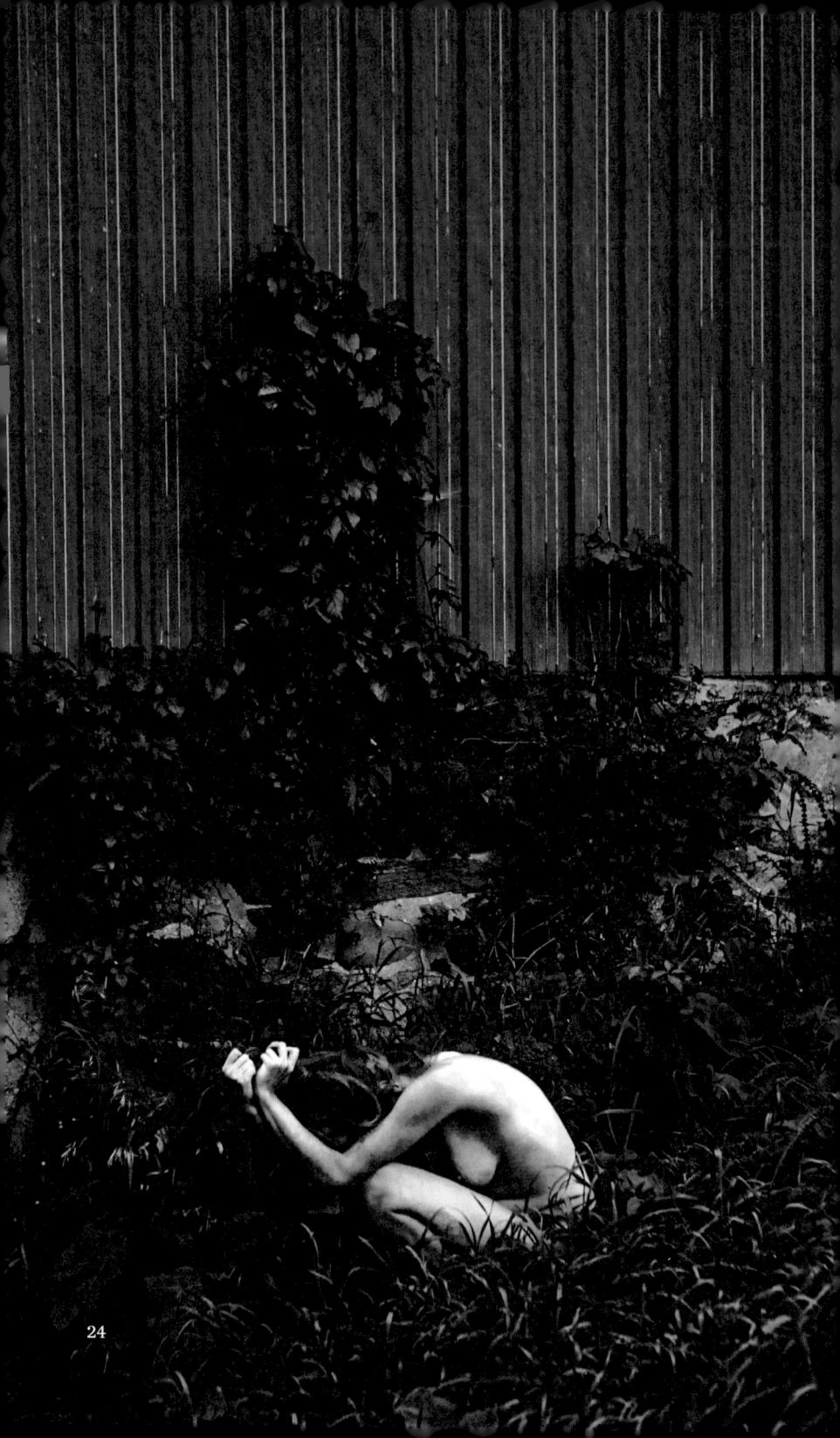

ANABELA PIERSOL

is full of surprises. Most folks will recognize her as the creative mind behind Fieldguided—a blog and brand known best for well-designed tote bags featuring lyrics by Kate Bush and David Bowie. Despite her Instagram-bred notoriety, Anabela is humble and down-to-earth. Since becoming a mom, self care has new meaning. She submitted the first draft of this essay before her son was born, and made a few revisions after entering motherhood — and realizing that being a parent is like being a passenger on an airplane adhering to safety procedures: You're supposed to apply your own oxygen mask before assisting the person next to you. In other words, you can't properly care for someone else until you're okay being you.

These Days
by Anabela Piersol

When I was dumped by my therapist, what I needed most was to feel safe. That year, the hits kept coming. I had experienced three miscarriages that broke my heart, and I no longer felt very sure-footed as I tried to navigate the world. I didn't need to feel safe from the usual hazards to one's health and well-being, but rather safe from conversations or images that cropped up like landmines and would cause me to start crying in public. I clung desperately to people that made me feel safe (literally: I know the sensation of gripping my husband's arm so well), and I ventured only to places on an approved list I kept filed away in my head. I withdrew from most of my friends, I had social media-induced panic attacks. I had to negotiate the world without a guide, despite how fragile I felt. I revisited Dante for the first time since university and wished I had a friend like Beatrice, who would be my advocate and help get me back on the right path. I thought about getting her words tattooed on my shoulder, *amor mi mosse, che mi fa parlare,* hoping that someone in the heavens would notice and intercede on my behalf. I felt frantic all the time. I found solace in what seemed to me to be the most unlikely places.

From January 2014 to the following January, I experienced recurrent miscarriages at about nine weeks each. This led to invasive tests of all sorts, and no answers to so many questions. During the second pregnancy, I visited a fertility clinic for a routine ultrasound, and I was told that the strong, tiny heartbeat that had been fluttering on the screen two weeks before was no longer there. Moments before, on a smaller screen in my hand, I had opened Facebook to see that someone had posted an ultrasound photo of her baby who would arrive a few months later. Although I had felt momentarily hopeless after the first miscarriage, my hope for a future filled with onesies and baby bottles had been quickly renewed. Now that bright vision was gone, and a hollow, empty feeling took its place. The ultrasound technician threw her arms around me and said she was sorry, but I wanted to disappear. Two days later I returned for a procedure that would remove the dead fetus from my body. I gripped my husband Geoff's hand and cried as we waited for my turn in the operating room. A nurse handed me an Ativan and said, "You think this is the worst thing that has ever happened to you, but it's not."

I had never thought of myself as a person who needed therapy. I wasn't clinically depressed, I thought, and I didn't see the value in therapy. After all, therapists are only human, and they only know as much as you tell them. But in late 2013, Geoff and I decided to see one. We both felt stuck in our professional lives and thought that maybe some outside help could nudge us in the right direction. We were willing to try anything. We met a therapist we liked and saw her for months. We built up a trust. After my two miscarriages, the focus shifted a little; I got used to sobbing in front of her. Once, after seeing her for about a year, I had called her to say that I was feeling down. She had always encouraged me to call or email her, saying that it was part of what I paid for, but I never did. So I called, and while sitting on a bench in the library where I work, I heard her say, "You like to feel sorry for yourself." "Pardon?" I said. "It's not like you live in Syria," she said. The sting was immediate: here was a trained professional telling me what I had been most afraid to hear: That I didn't deserve therapy because I didn't have real problems. She might as well have said, "Get over it, and get over yourself."

I was taken aback, and eventually channelled all my most hateful feelings towards her. How dare she? Even if she thought that about me, couldn't she have kept it to herself and maintained some kind of facade of professionalism? Had she thought that, about me, from the beginning? I told Geoff that I didn't want to see her again, but he went to see her alone and told her I was upset with her. We went to one final, tense appointment together where she talked only about herself. She didn't seem to remember what she had said, and told us she couldn't see us anymore. She could recommend other therapists. But from then on, I decided I was done with therapists. I had my third miscarriage a few months later, but by then I was on my own. My life felt out of control, and so I had to take control somehow, or retreat further into a dark place.

I had been slowly alienating myself from many of my friends. I couldn't talk to anyone who had a baby because I was afraid I wouldn't be able to contain my jealousy. I didn't want to feel jealous, which seemed like a hateful reaction to something lovely. The guilt felt just as painful. At the same time, I was grateful for those feelings because they reassured me that I really wanted a baby. I had been open about my first miscarriage, to the point of writing about it on my blog, but felt too afraid to talk about subsequent ones. I was deeply afraid of becoming everyone's "infertile friend." I didn't want to acknowledge that there was a possibility I would never be able to maintain a pregnancy. If I talked about it, maybe the spark of hope would fade. I certainly didn't want people to think I liked feeling sorry for myself, lest I hear: "At least you don't live in Syria," again. If someone mentioned surrogacy or adoption, I would break down, because they seemed like impossible alternatives. I thought about starting a casual support group with like-minded women going through similar difficulties. So many women suffer through infertility and pregnancy loss, I learned, as women quietly reached out to me. I thought about writing about my experiences so these women wouldn't feel alone. But I never did. Besides, I hadn't had my happy ending, and who wants to read a story without one, I thought. It was an incredibly lonely time.

I started seeing a naturopath. I began downing fistfuls of supplements. I consulted online forums (but only briefly, as I could only handle so much before clicking away nervously). I created a yoga room in my apartment and carried healing crystals in my pocket which I charged in the light of the full moon. I focused all my energy on feeling safe, and that took on the (admittedly strange) shape of visiting specific places. There were certain unlikely places that made me feel calm, even if they were busy and bustling: Boutique gyms around the city, using a pass that gave me access to as many as I wanted to visit; the Pacific Mall, a suburban mall filled with, among other things, counterfeit goods imported from China; the Canadian National Exhibition, a fair that visits Toronto for a few weeks in August; and the Sunnyside Pool, one of the busier pools in downtown Toronto that looks out to Lake Ontario.

It's hard to explain why these places and unlikely pastimes were so important to me during some of the hardest moments of my life. Riding my bike across town to get to a ballet-inspired fitness class where I spun around in circles, or to a kickboxing class where I clobbered a rubber dummy with my fists; Surrounded by strangers, I could feel strong and graceful, even if I knew, and even if the mirrors in front of me, told me I wasn't, not really. I would run through ravines and shady trails and every kilometre I logged was a triumph, although I never tallied up more than I could count on one hand. Wandering around the mall and looking at fake Moschino rubber phone cases and eating cheap hand-pulled noodles made me feel calm. In the bustle of the CNE I never worried about bumping into anyone I knew, although I still gripped Geoff's arm tightly.

> *I had been slowly alienating myself from many of my friends. I couldn't talk to anyone who had a baby, because I was afraid I wouldn't be able to contain my jealousy.*

I was just one of thousands of strangers. The rides, which have always felt so rickety and ready to fall apart at any moment, gave me a momentary feeling of euphoria. I loved the overwhelming greasy smells of blooming onions and deep-fried funnel cake batter.

I would go to the pool with one particular body-positive friend who had never been too interested in discussing reproduction, and was therefore, in my mind, safe to be around. At the pool I would spend the first ten minutes applying sunscreen, then enter the cool water. I would close my eyes and float on my back and feel the sun on my eyelids, making everything go white. The sounds of shouting and splashing would be muffled. It's the closest you can feel to not having a body, and my body had given me so much trouble.

Maybe that was the trick: these places somehow gave me an otherworldly feeling, and I didn't have to talk to anyone, therapist or otherwise, to get there. The preceding months had left me wilted and weak. I thought I was useless. But after a good workout or a run, that momentary high of feeling powerful for even a few moments was one that I chased. Travelling to the Pacific Mall is a bit of a hike, enough to make one feel very far away. At the mall I would walk from one shop to another which sold items identical to the last, drinking a bubble tea, and I felt as though I was somewhere faraway. I had only gone to the CNE twice as a child, and both of those times are mythologized in my memory; maybe I was recapturing the feeling of being a kid again, a kid with no real responsibilities. The pool made me feel weightless and free.

> *I was recapturing the feeling of being a kid again, a kid with no real responsibilities. The pool made me feel weightless and free.*

Ultimately, these were my ways of coping. They weren't a cure for my sadness and the methods weren't surefire, either. I went to the CNE on what would have been the due date of my first pregnancy, August 24. I had been haunted by that date, putting so much meaning on it: the loss of my hope. I went to the CNE deliberately to try to forget it. I walked around the grounds with Geoff, my brother, and my sister-in-law, and felt the persistent melancholic twinge that lingered behind the happiness I found in the bright lights. My brother won an oversized stuffed doughnut in a shooting game and gave it to me. I made a slow-motion video on my phone of the swings titling and flying high above as the sun faded behind the horizon, and my sister-in-law said, "Look how happy she is."

As I write this, I have my sleeping infant next to me in a Moses basket. He's eight weeks old, and I can't keep from reaching over from time to time to stroke his soft leg or to neurotically check his breathing. The love I feel for him overwhelms me at times. Ironically, I was diagnosed with postpartum depression and have started counselling. No matter how much I yearned for this baby, no matter how complete I feel, I know that depression is a terrifying beast that will find me. And that what worked for me once before won't work again. Maybe I have managed to heal what had been broken, but in the process, I've softened my once-firm stance against seeking help. I don't want to go at it alone, because this time, it's not just about me.

"VICKY LAM, JEN SPINNER AND CHRISTINA YAN

will find the time to make personal work that matters to them. Even if that means they might only have energy left to make cereal for dinner. All three work full-time as commercial artists in their chosen field — Vicky as a photographer, Jen as an art director and Christina as a stylist. They stretch themselves to create work outside of their day jobs because it nourishes them.

The concept for these still lifes started as a conversation between friends. When did they feel most joyful about food? Burdened by it? When did making or eating food symbolize bigger needs — to fuel up, be cared for, celebrate, or treat themselves?

The work explores a range of food-related experiences shared by all three collaborators. Such as, feeling grateful for the fresh groceries in the fridge. Or, resisting feeling guilty about having no time to make an elaborate breakfast. Self care means allowing yourself the space to make the choices that are right for you — and understanding that "what's right" is always subject to change.

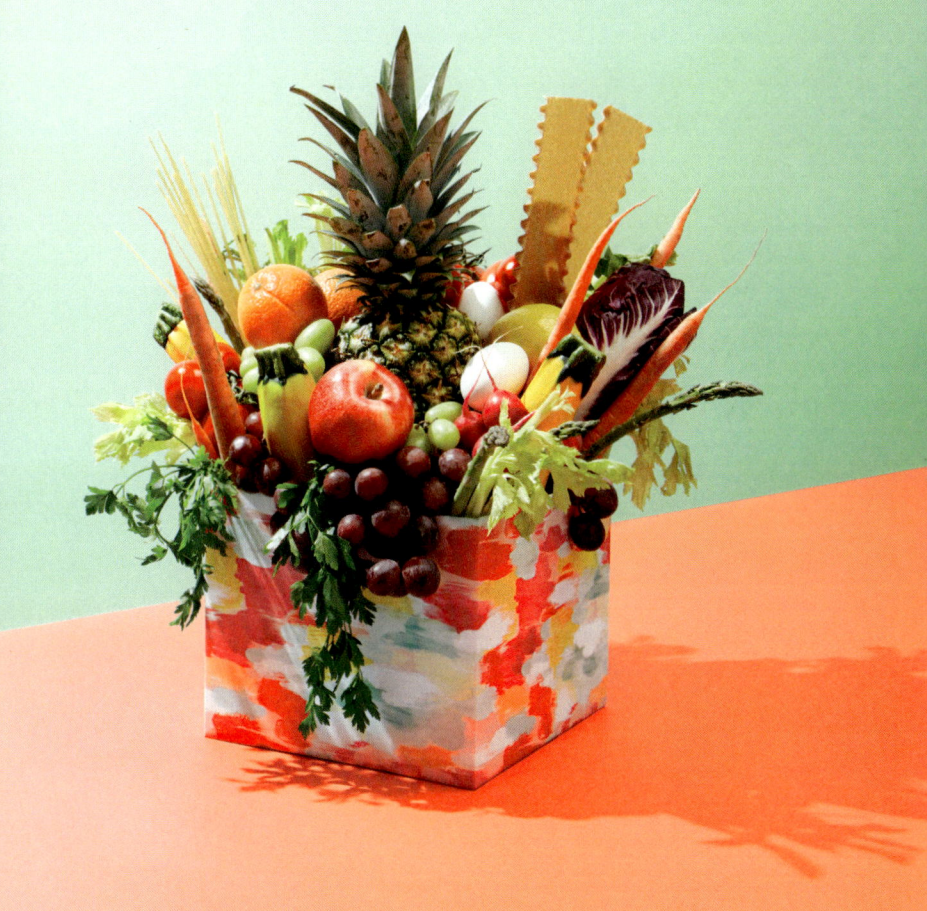

VICKY LAM, JEN SPINNER & CHRISTINA YAN
THE STUFF THAT FEEDS US

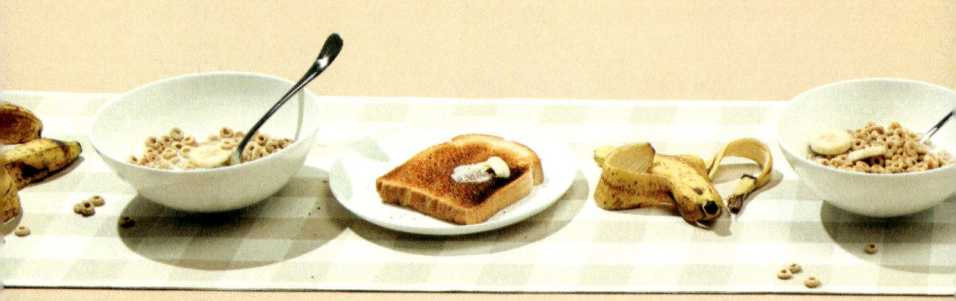

YOU CARE TOO MUCH

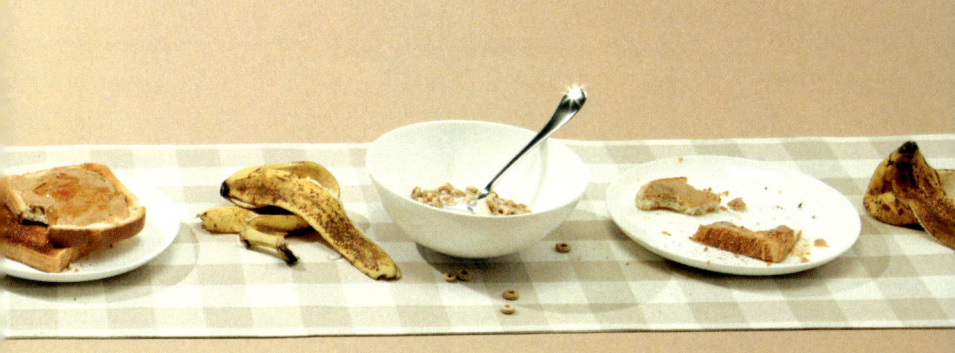

VICKY LAM, JEN SPINNER & CHRISTINA YAN
THE STUFF THAT FEEDS US

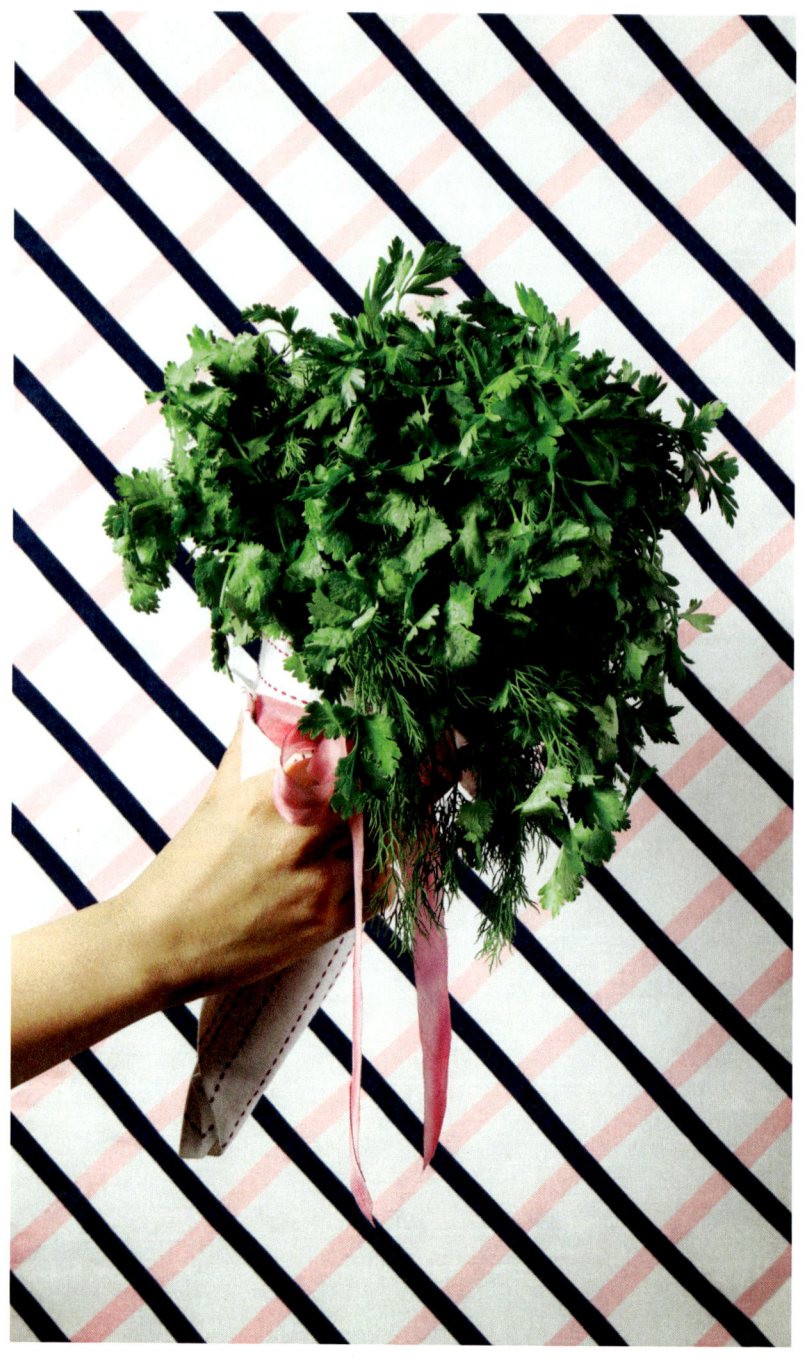

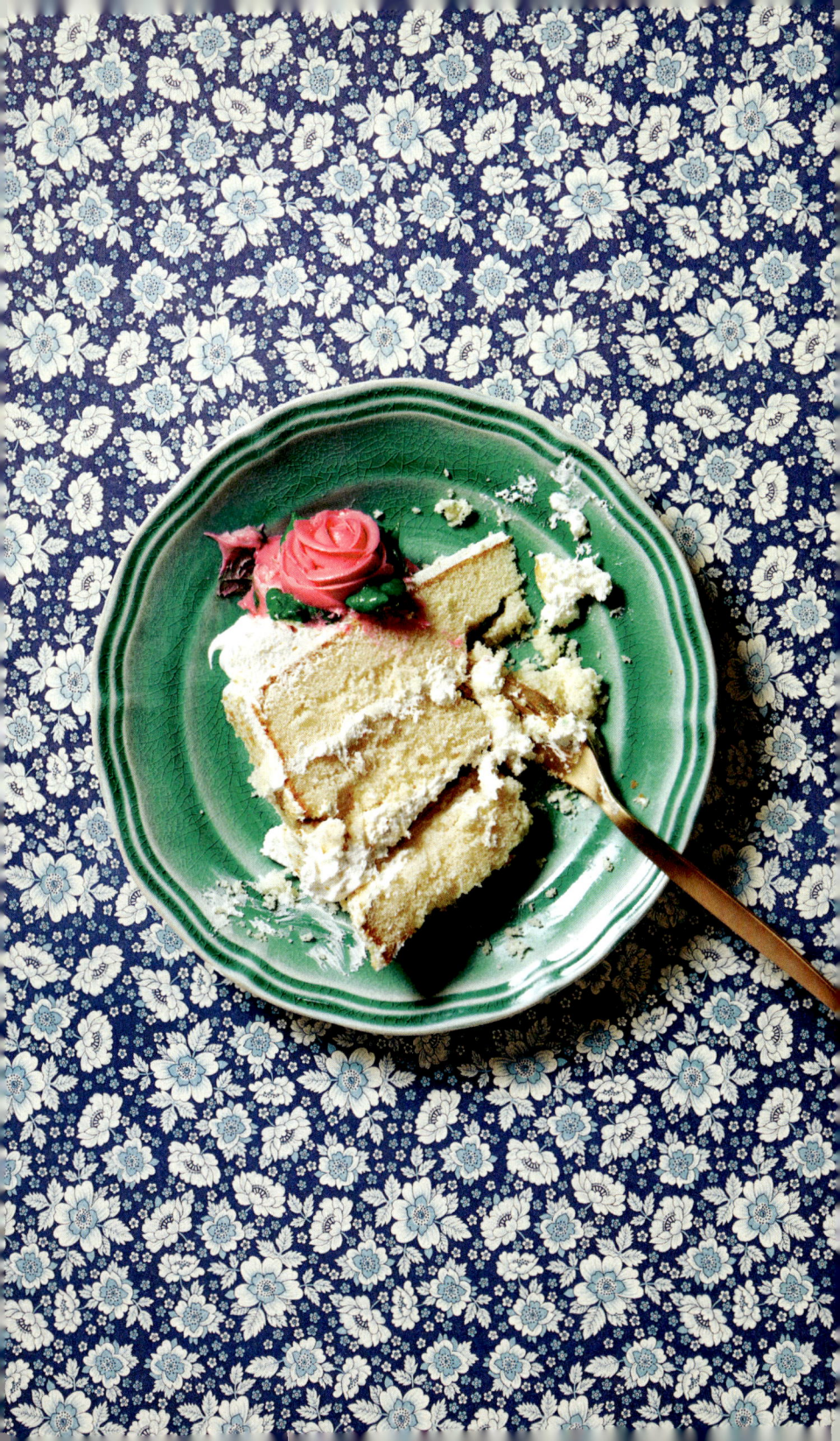

WINNIE TRUONG

gives herself space to make mistakes. She describes her studio as a fluid and creative space that allows her to mentally and physically make things, but also gives her the freedom to fail. After all, great art often comes from taking risks.

Winnie lives and works in Toronto, where she received a BFA from the Ontario College of Art and Design's drawing and painting program. In the spirit of new experiences and bold shifts, her paper cut drawings came about during a two month stint at Fool's Paradise, Doris McCarthy's Artist-in-Residence program. These selections, from a larger body of work, are complex and emotionally challenging — and ask us to think about our heavily coded ideas of nature and femininity.

Winnie brings to life a female subject that is all at once fragile, robust, and blasé. Playing with the parallels between anatomy and botany, grooming and landscaping, these wimmin subvert all physical and biological possibilities by birthing their own environments and thus emphasizing the female body as a wellspring of endless creation, expression and transgression.

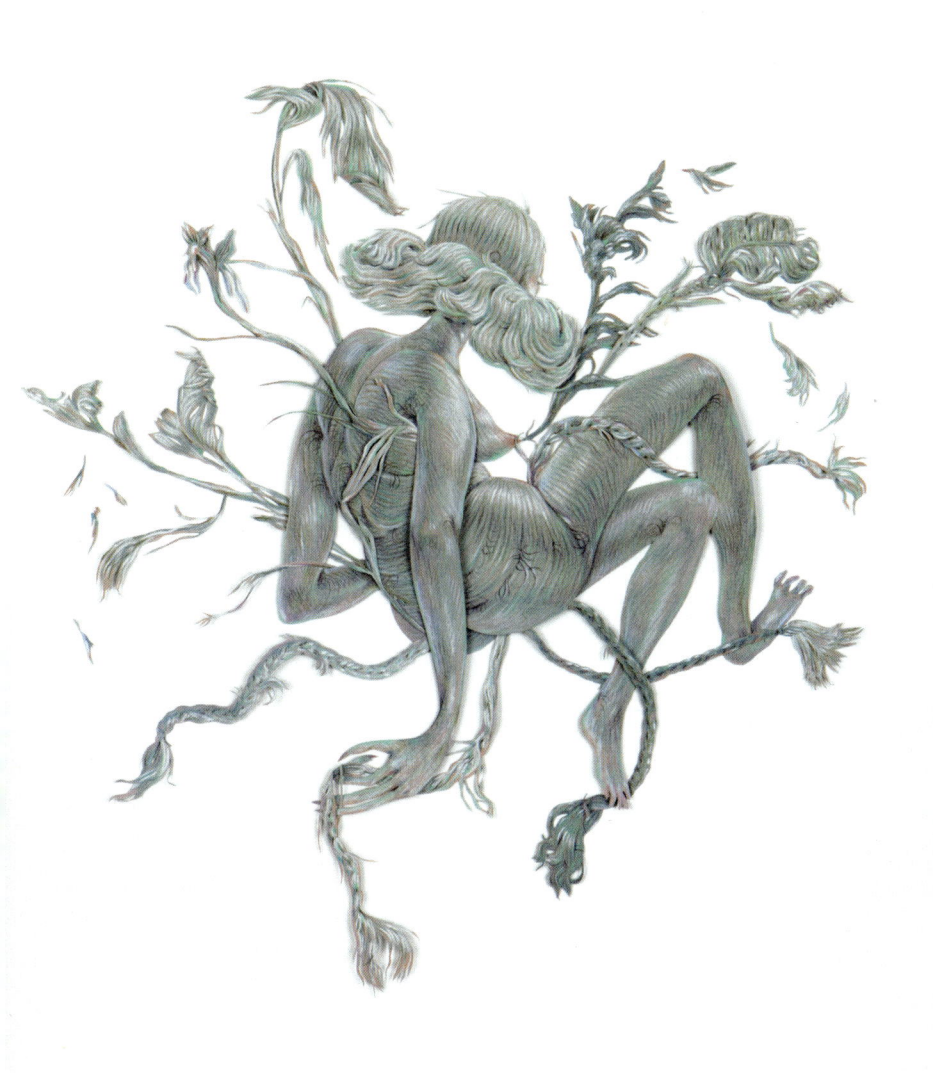

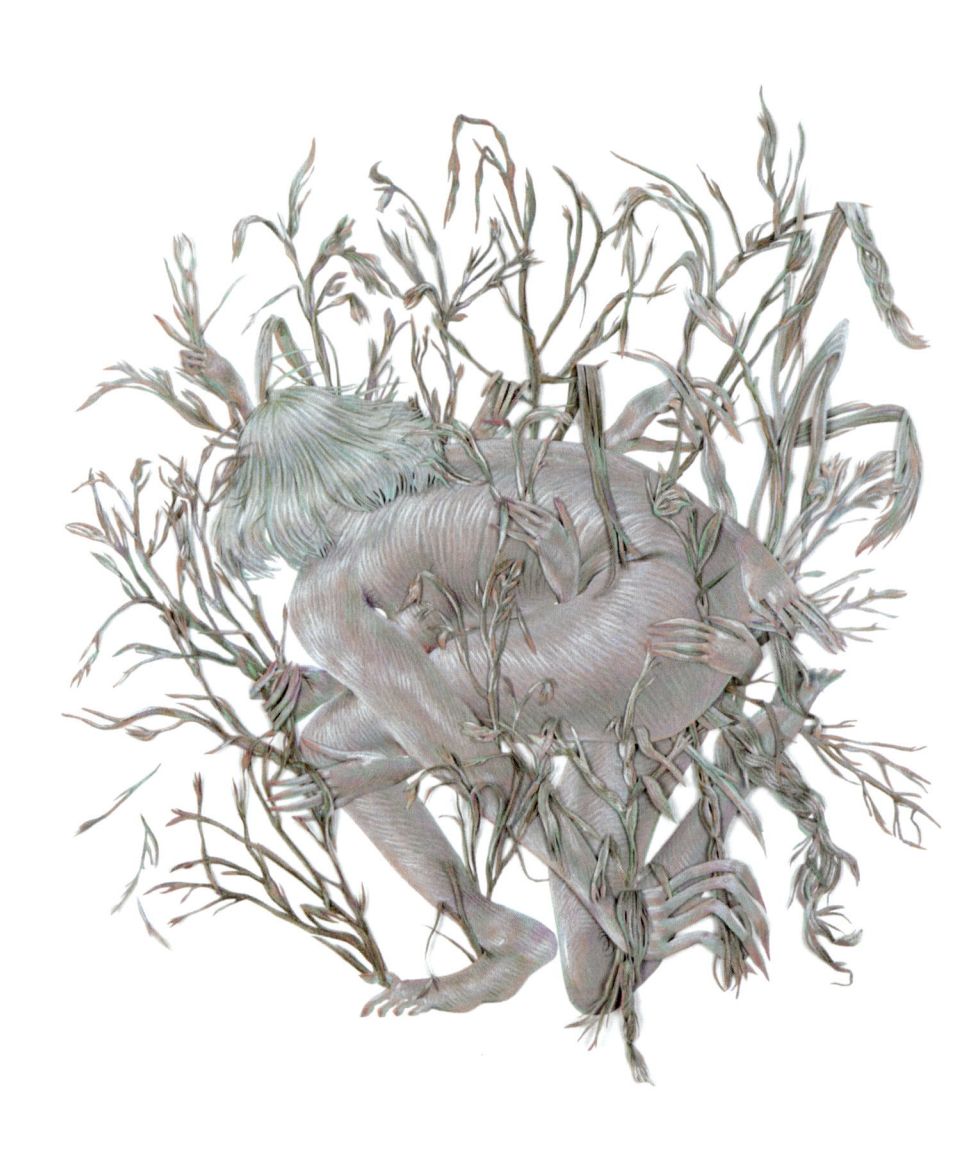

Each intricate piece in Winnie's **Paper Cut** *series on pages 39–43 is created with coloured pencil on cut paper.*

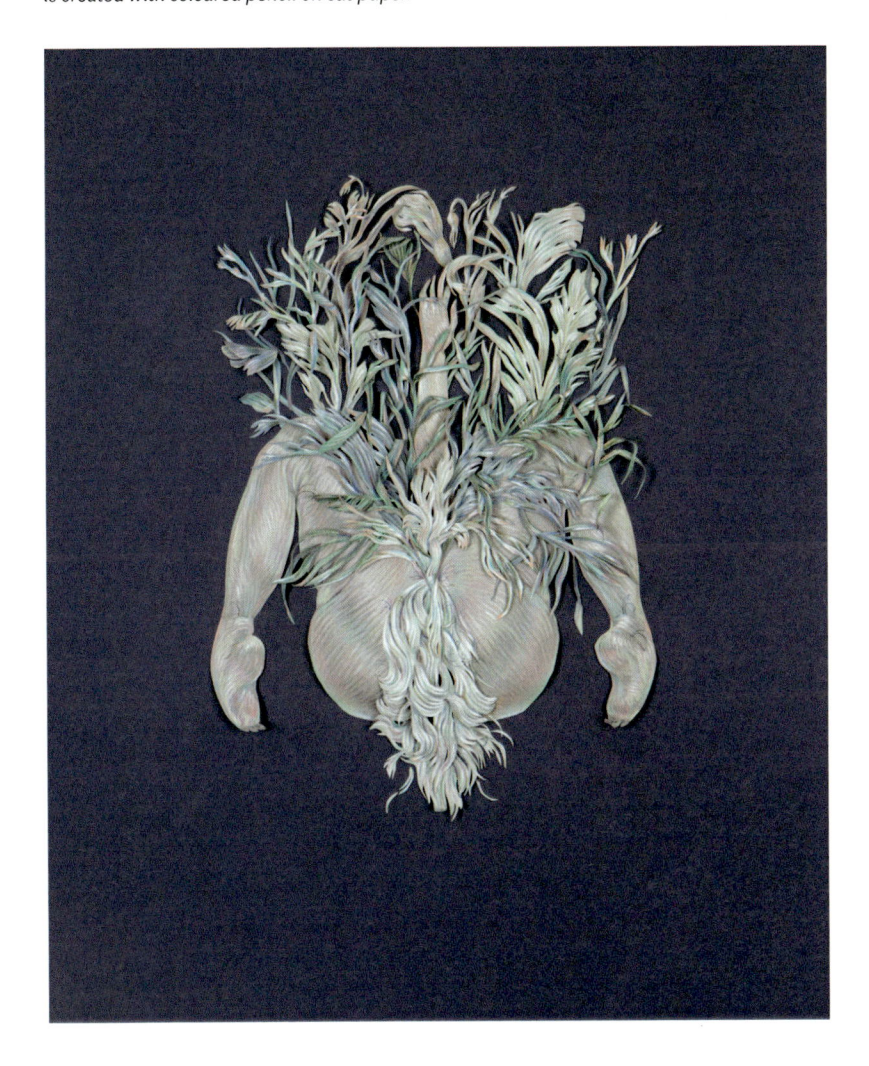

WINNIE TRUONG / PAPER CUTS, FIVE FINGERED BOUQUET

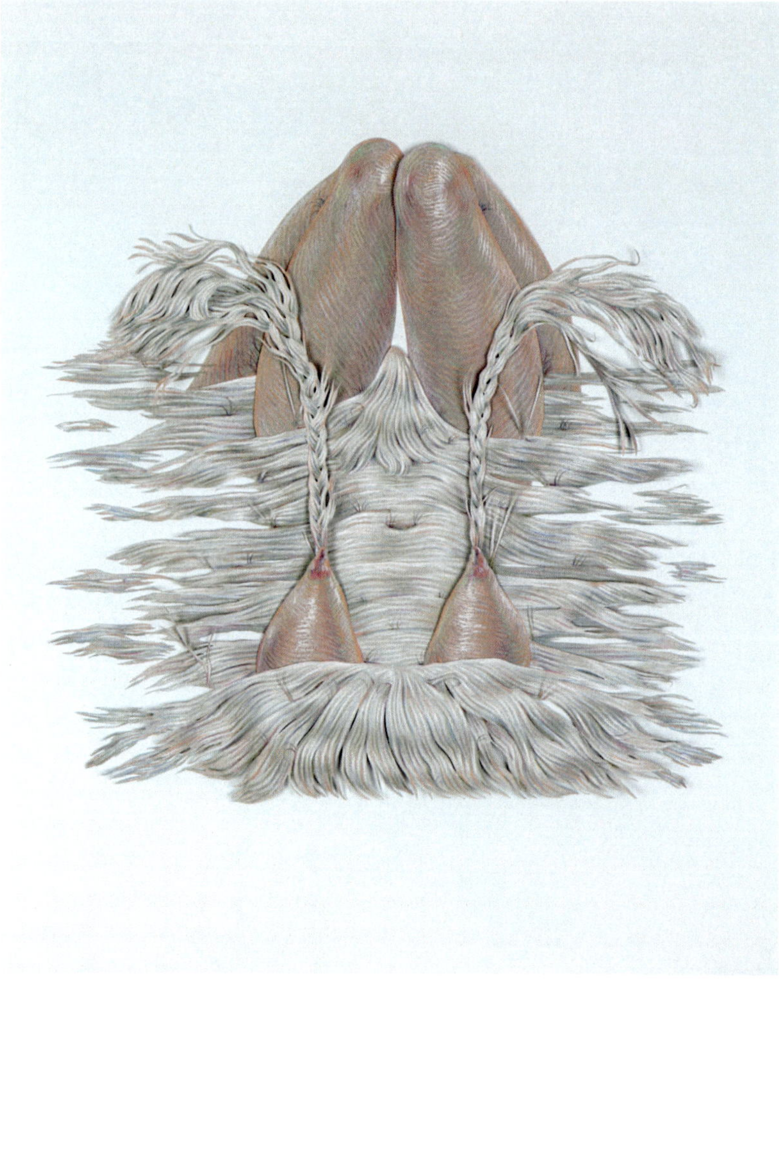

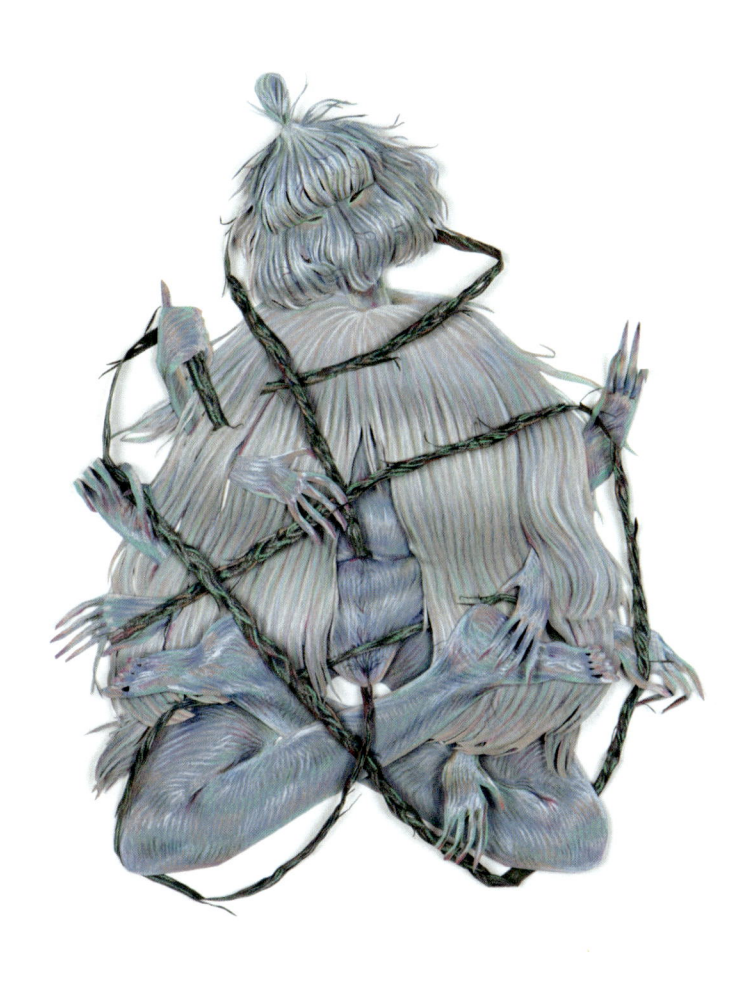

Feelings can be art.

without pretend

/wɪðˈaʊt, wɪθ-/ /prɪˈtɛnd/
(idiom.)

1. An act of bravery; a way of living which is free from pretense; a state of being achieved between feats of fantastic strength and moments spent searching, wondering, and wishing for more.

2. An independent publisher focused on producing, promoting and distributing works by female-identifying writers and visual artists who make thoughtful, meaningful work.

Origin: 2015; Toronto, Ontario, Canada

withoutpretend.com

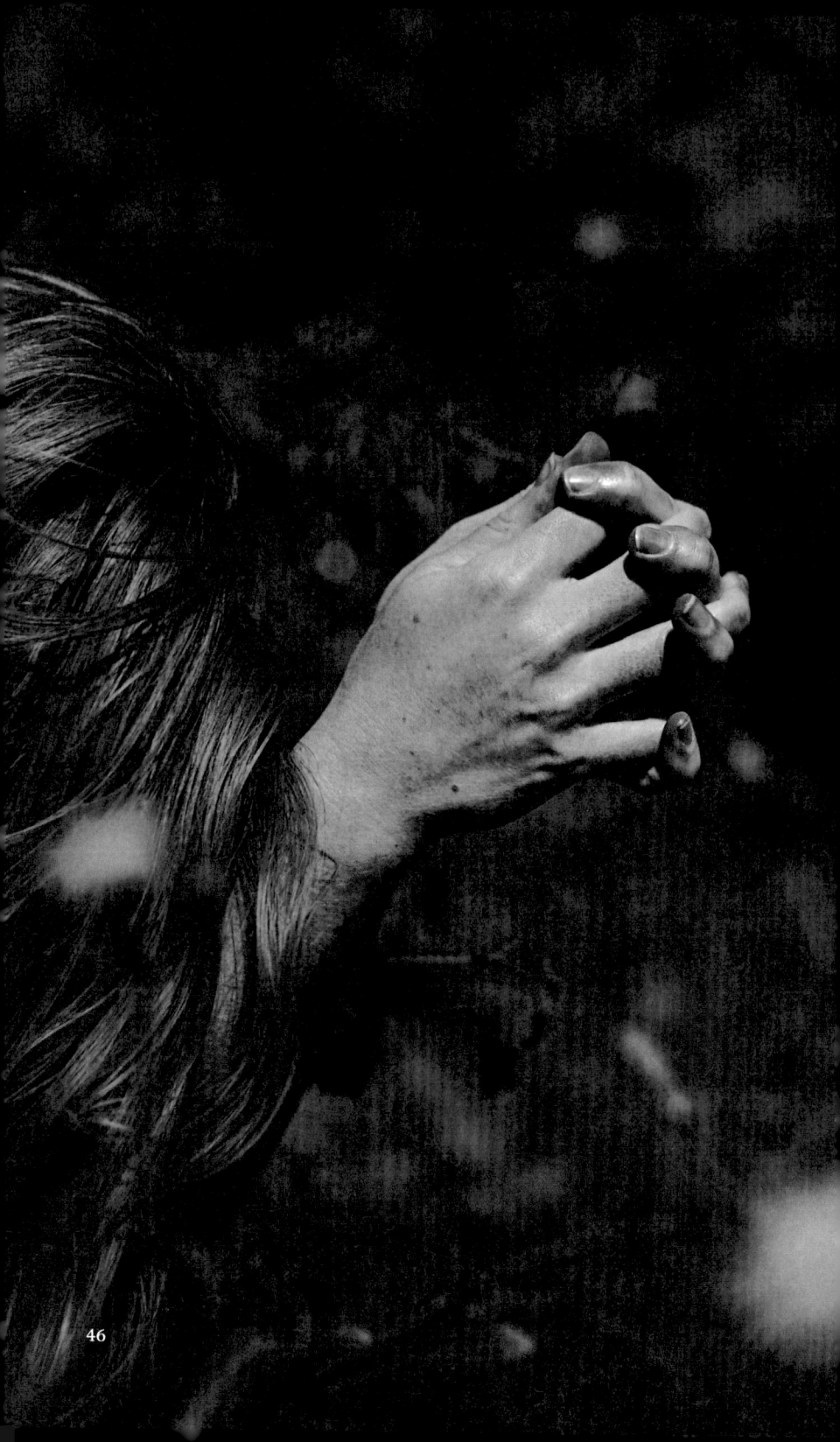

SOFIA MOSTAGHIMI

sees the world in stories. Born in Sherbrooke, Quebec, but raised in the Greater Toronto Area, Sofia is inspired to write stories about ordinary places and the people that are marked by them. Her short story for this collection is about a young woman coping with the death of her father, and self care is presented as a process of internal reflection — about carving out an identity in relation to her family, friends, romantic interests and the world at large. Sofia earned her masters in creative writing in Toronto where she now lives and teaches high school English. She is currently working on completing her first novel, *Claire and Caen*.

Fall in Love if You're So Unhappy

by Sofia Mostaghimi

I heard bombs from my bed. I lived in Toronto, working on Bloor Street in the backroom of an expensive furniture store. I stocked shelves. I repriced merchandise. Humanity burned my eyes. That was a pain that I'd always had, and when my mom called me in the evenings, and asked me what was wrong, I told her about what I'd seen, almost against my will, on TV. I told her Israel. I told her Palestine. Syria. Venezuela. The United States of America. I told her ISIS and the Highway of Tears and the killing of unarmed black youth. She'd cluck that Middle-Eastern sound of disapproval she'd learned to make against the roof of her mouth from watching my paternal grandmother, and say that my dad immigrated here for a reason.

"You have the luxury of not having to concern yourself with these things. You are Canadian."

Yet the fate of the mixed-raced baby is the dilemma of in-betweens. I am Canadian and I am not. I am white and I am brown. "I don't have your luxury," I'd tell her. I can't be either and I can't be both. I am all things and I am nothing.

My brother's voice still crept inside of my head:

"Shut up."

"Get over yourself."

"You're one of the lucky ones."

Daniel still had his life together then: the blonde, symmetrical girlfriend; the corner unit of a glass condo with a linen closet; the All But Dissertation — All But Disappointment, my brother. If I'd wanted, I could have gone back to school, too and done a Master's in something. My grades had been good. Instead, I told my mom that I wished I hadn't ever gone to university, that I had lived a different version of freedom.

"What's wrong with you?" Daniel would call just to shout at me. "Why do you have to say things like that to her? Especially now. It's not Mom's fault if you can't get your shit together. Fall in love if you're so unhappy. At least for a little while that'll help."

He meant like our parents had. Stubborn star-crossed lovers that, against all odds, had lived the happily-ever-after—until, of course, he died.

"He isn't *white*," my mom told me one night on the phone. "When I walked down the street with your dad that's all I was thinking. That when people saw us holding hands, they weren't seeing two people in love. They were seeing an interracial couple. A white woman with a brown man. My God, that's heavy for a twenty-three year old if you stop and think about it, just walking down the street. Like we were, I don't know, making a political statement. It's only looking back now that I understand it as that though. At the time, how I framed it with your dad was just, he isn't *white* and I am. I felt so guilty for thinking that. Because it wasn't even my voice. It was—I don't know. But thank God for love, and look how beautifully you and your brother turned out."

The stories about my father made me sad. I had never considered myself a pessimist, but I could feel myself becoming one. I was angrier, almost fatalistic. So I took up my brother's advice and decided that I was going to fall in love. Having never been in love, I prayed to the gods of Beginner's Luck. I cried myself to sleep a lot, too, which was maybe a way to summon them. If I still couldn't sleep I'd walk the long hallway of my one bedroom apartment past the bathroom, into my small, square kitchen that always smelled faintly of tahini from the shawarma shop below, and sit and stare at Amélie Poulain, the famous weirdo from that French movie and the eternal insomniac inside of my glossy poster. All day she sat trapped underneath the turquoise covers of her bed, flipping through photographs with this half-bent smile that I couldn't figure out. It was during one of those early mornings while I stared at Amélie Poulain that I noticed I had a roommate: small, grey, and nimble, that slipped frantically through the crack between the oven and countertop at the slightest sound of me. A mouse.

I'd hear the thing in the walls, too, or see it scurry across the kitchen floor when the light from the hallway came on automatically. It ate through all of my pasta packages in the pantry, and broke into a bag of lentils. On my worst nights, when I'd try to fall asleep, I'd imagine its sole purpose was to make me nervous for the privilege I'd unjustly inherited in this life.

For the next few days, I thought about laying mouse traps: under the oven, behind the refrigerator. Instead, I named her Rosy and talked incessantly about her to my mom. How she'd come nibble at bits of wet food in the sink, or how I could hear her squeaking sometimes, but I didn't know why and I wished I did.

The following weekend, my mom had Daniel drop off a bag of traps.

"I don't know why you can't buy your own fucking mouse traps," he'd said standing on my back deck. He was shivering in a leather jacket and dark jeans. Under his eyes were bags, yellow and puffy.

"Are you sleeping okay?" I'd asked him.

"Fine," he'd said.

He wouldn't come inside. I tried handing him the money for the traps but he wouldn't take it. He said he and Vanessa were thinking about going to Mexico soon. He wanted to see if he could get rid of the cold he couldn't seem to shake. Then he said he had to go. He was late. I watched him from my back deck drive away too fast to be safe.

Inside, I opened the bag of traps on the kitchen table. I took out some cheese. I took the traps out of the bags. But I physically couldn't bring myself to set them.

It was obvious to me even then: I wanted to occupy this in-between space, one where I could live without the blame of having killed, or of knowing that I was a coward.

I toyed with unlikely fantasies during this time. I meet an attractive man at a bus stop. We marry and move to a new house (where there is no mouse). A fire ignites in the furniture store where I work and a firefighter saves me then woos me. An attractive man places a toonie into a homeless man's cup at the very same time as I do, our fingers touch; he asks me out on a date, offers to set the bait in my traps for me. Attractive man and me meet elsewhere: the bookstore, the airport lounge, the airplane, the streetcar, the line for a co-ed washroom, the pharmacy, the grocery store, the coffee shop where the lattes come with swans and happy faces foamed on top, all those places, really, that I never go.

His name was Victor. We met unromantically by swiping right instead of left on each other's profile pictures. It was my last remaining friend, Golnar, who told me about the app, installed it for me, and swiped for an hour on my behalf because she said I was being too picky. Amélie Poulain watched us at my kitchen table while the sun set through the window above my pyramid of dirty dishes. She watched as Golnar also spilled red wine into her cleavage, caught her fingers inside the mouse traps several times as she set them, laughed hysterically for the duration of a burp then said that if I didn't get rid of Rosy soon fat mouse-babies would start to populate my apartment until our fates became intertwined and I disappeared into the thick of them.

"What the hell does that mean?" I asked.

"You never heard of a Rat King?"

"No."

"It's when a bunch of rodents living together in a small space get their tails knotted together so then they become one giant rodent. Their feces is like, the glue. They develop herd mentality. It's called a Rat King."

"You're actually disgusting."

"It's a real, scientific thing, so you better watch out."

Golnar pulled up a photo of a Rat King on her phone. I told her I didn't want to see it, but she insisted. The image was of the brown dried up corpses of rats with their dark tails tangled, and their stiff bodies overtop of one another, fanned out to make the shape of a haphazard circle. She laughed, looking at me look at the photo.

How many people had died from diseases carried by these creatures? And what sort of condition was this, even for a rodent? For any living thing?

"Oh please," she'd said. "Do not get over-analytical here." She always had a way of knowing where my thoughts were going. She took her phone back and picked mine up from the edge of the table. She told me she was going to get me laid for the sake of my sanity, but also our friendship. A few minutes later, a dating app had been installed on my phone, and Golnar was laughing again, sifting through pictures of me to set up my profile.

"Doesn't the fact that this app has to exist depress the hell out of you, Golnar?"

Golnar looked up from my phone and moved her free hand to set overtop of mine. She smiled, "It's okay to admit you're lonely."

Just then Rosy peeked out from between her favourite crack near the oven, and Golnar screamed. She folded her legs up to her chest on the chair, and yelled for it to go away.

"See, I'm not lonely. I've got Rosy," I said.

Rosy disappeared and Golnar's scream turned into a laugh, loud and horrifying.

"Oh my God," she exclaimed. "How do you sleep at night? I wouldn't sleep at night!"

When Golnar was finally calm she thanked me for letting her drink all of my wine. She put my phone back into my hand. She said not to be so hard on all the boys I was going to meet, and to always use a condom, and to remember while I watched the news that there was a little contraption called the TV remote that could make it all go away.

"That's the thing though," I told her. "It doesn't all go away."

"Get laid," she'd said. Then she left, very drunk, into a cab.

Victor messaged me hello the next day. He said I looked pretty in my pictures, especially the one where I glanced sideways at the sky. I told him I'd done that on purpose, so that the picture would look more candid. He laughed virtually with a haha then asked me what my background was. I asked him what his background was. Golnar told me once that answering a question with another question was an easy way of seeming coy and flirtatious. He told me to guess then sent another haha. I told him I didn't like to guess. We changed the subject.

I told him about Rosy. He told me he'd once had a cockroach infestation in his first apartment downtown, and how he'd learned that cockroaches can survive a nuclear blast, and they will eat soap if no real food is available, or even each other if they have to. He told me to be thankful it wasn't cockroaches; so I told my mom I was thankful Rosy wasn't a cockroach on the phone later that week. She asked me where this sudden, small burst of optimism was coming from. She was excited when I told her about Victor.

"I remember when I first met your dad," my mom's voice shuddered when she spoke of him. "We were at an engagement party. We'd both come alone and I noticed him as soon as I walked in. Well, not as soon as I walked in—when I went into the kitchen to fetch a vase for the flowers I'd brought. But then later, when we'd all had a bit too much to drink, your dad came up to me with this little snippet of a white flower he cut from a bouquet and he gave it to me. My God. I was laughing so hard, I was almost crying, because it was a flower from the bouquet I brought. He was re-gifting my flower to me. Anyway, the beginning is nice. The beginning is so sweet. Enjoy it," she said. "But you didn't say. Where did you guys meet?"

I couldn't think of anything to say, and Rosy was making noise in the pantry.

"He's an exterminator," I said.

"Oh," she said.

"But I think he wants to go back to school."

I could hear her breathing then suddenly she was laughing.

"Isn't it so funny how certain situations lead us to just the right people?"

Later that night, my brother called to ask if the mouse was dead yet.

"You mean, Rosy?" I asked.

I should have known that when he shouted about what an idiot I was for naming the thing or, for that matter, working at a furniture store when I had an Honours Bachelors in Science, that it wasn't really about me at all.

"Do you think Dad came to Canada for you to do something so meaningless? For you to be so insignificant?" he asked.

When I hung up the phone, I was crying. I had four unread messages. Three from Victor, two of which were composed entirely out of food emojis, and one from Golnar, which read: Bang anyone yet? ;)

Victor and I met in person two weeks later. I'd already decided that when I introduced him to my mom we were going to say that we met through my landlord who'd agreed to have an exterminator come take a look at my apartment. We'd say that I'd forgotten anyone was coming when I heard a knock at my door. I had just gotten out of the shower and my hair was wet when we first met. Then we'd laugh as we told our lie and my mom would laugh too. We'd say it was love at first sight. And isn't it funny how everything happens for a reason? Victor was only working as an exterminator temporarily while he waited to see if he got into med school, which he had and was going to attend in September.

It was only when the real Victor sat across from me in an empty bar at 5 p.m. that I realized I hadn't ever actually asked him what he did. I wasn't sure if I even cared. There'd been another mass shooting in the States, and Syrian refugees were cold and dying of starvation while ISIS continued its trafficking of Yazidi women. Behind the bar where we'd each ordered our pints before choosing a table near the window, was a skinny, bored girl with blue hair and tattoos folding cutlery into napkins that Victor kept glancing over my head at while we talked.

Victor was different than I thought he would be. His shoulders sloped. He smiled more than an adult should, like the whole world was a big joke. And he thought Toronto was only an "OK city," and that London and Dubai was where better things were happening.

> *Victor was different than I thought he would be. His shoulders sloped. He smiled more than an adult should, like the whole world was a big joke.*

"Some people put their dicks up as profile pics," he said, smiling, "and your tag line was 'contact only if interested in falling in love.'"

"I know. I posted it," I said.

"You don't think it's a bit weird to go looking for love on a one-night stand app?"

He'd already gulped down half of his beer.

"No."

I asked him if he followed the news and if he had seen all the protests that were happening.

"Don't you know you shouldn't talk about politics on a first date?" he asked.

A red streetcar drummed against the tracks outside the window. We listened to it pass.

"I don't care if the things that matter make you feel uncomfortable," I said.

The bartender seemed to have choked on air and was wheezing and coughing behind us. We heard the tap, the sound of water gushing into a glass. Victor stared at me. He seemed to be concentrating very hard on not smiling.

At my place, we both sat on my bed. Victor told me things like we were in a "solar maximum" year which is where every eleven years the sun gets louder and a bit hotter; that the way a bee colony chooses their new members is that they have a few bees feed on royal jelly as larvae then fight to the death as adults; that St. Patrick's Day was illegal to celebrate in Toronto as recently as thirty years ago because the Irish gathering in large groups was considered a threat bordering on terrorism; that romantic love, in the way that we view it, is a recent, nineteenth century construct popularized by novels.

"But what about *Romeo and Juliet*? That was written in the 1500s."

I sat diagonal to him. He was leaning against the wall instead of my headboard, with his legs spread out perfectly still in front of him. We had been kissing for a little bit, then paused the kissing to talk again.

"People didn't used to expect love to be the reason they'd marry," he said. "That's the difference."

"Are your parents divorced?"

"No. My mom was a refugee. She lost her first husband in the war then she met my dad here, and they had me," he said. He put his big, thick hand over my cheek to keep my head still as he leaned in again to kiss me. I pulled away.

"That explains a lot," I said.

His mom loved then lost. She remarried a new man for practical purposes.

"What?"

"Nothing," I said.

"Say it. I'm interested in knowing what you have to say."

"I have nothing to say," I said. I moved in to kiss him but he pushed my cheek away. When I looked at him again, he'd let the sides of his mouth fall.

"You think my views on love are skewed because of my personal experiences?" he asked. He laughed, "Which you know nothing about?"

"I just mean, I stock shelves for a living after graduating top of my class. My dad died suddenly for no reason. Those personal experiences have skewed my views."

"In what way?" he asked.

"In the way that everything sucks and I want to die."

Victor leaned forward with that body of his that I had already decided I was going to love, and he brought his hand up to my cheek and slapped it. He slapped me and the human tragedy of it reverberated in me, like people dying overseas, and everywhere in the streets. The world is just your backyard, my dad used to say. My head burned with his voice. The tears I tried to suppress were worms squirming to get out, pressing the underneath of where I caked concealer to hide my exhaustion.

This is your life, the slap said, loudly.

I caught my breath in deep inhales to try not to cry but I did anyway. I cried. Victor blinked. *Who is this guy?* I was thinking. *I don't even know you.* I screamed for him to get out. I think those were the words that were coming out of my mouth, for him just to leave.

"I don't even know you. I let you into my house. Get out!"

Those must have been the words I was saying because I could see the scared look in his eyes. I could feel the future we might have had receding back down into that abyss where lie all the souls of the innocent dead.

"I'm sorry," I think I heard him say. Suddenly, we were both standing in my kitchen by my back door, surrounded by so many empty mouse traps. He was slipping into his shoes which were polished and brown. "But you shouldn't say things like that. You should be more thankful. You don't say things like that."

By then I couldn't remember why he had slapped me. I felt only the humiliation and fear.

"Get out! Get out! Get out!"

He left and I never saw him again. In the silence of my apartment, I heard Rosy squirming behind a kitchen wall. I heard drywall crumbling as she shifted and made my walls her home. I walked to the bathroom and looked at my face in the mirror. I faked a smile. I caught mascara and tears with the sides of my fingers, and watched myself wipe them against my jeans. If my dad were still alive today he would have laughed and called me dramatic. So I did it for him. I laughed. I walked back into the kitchen, opened my refrigerator door, and got out a hunk of cheddar cheese, sobbing and laughing, and ate the whole fucking thing. A few days later, Rosy was dead, caught in a trap behind the radiator with a piece of cheese in her mouth and a broken neck. ◗

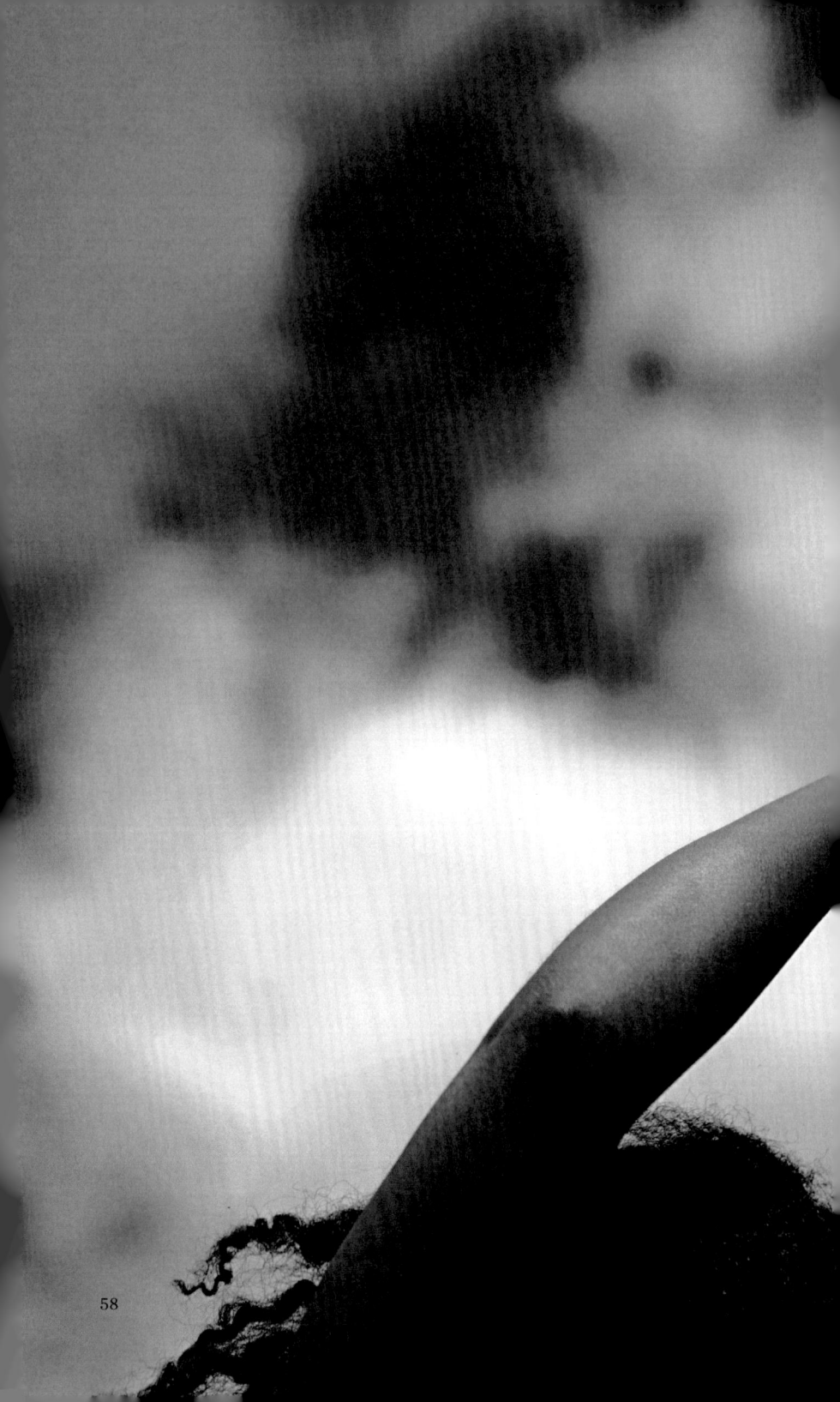

NAOMI MOYER

feels like she's on the right path. She's had to work hard to find that path, but now writes and makes art about the very things she grew up feeling most ashamed about. Naomi has been interested in the theme of self care for years, and the inspiration to write this essay about her left hand has been building up over time. Even though she has written and self-published an entire zine called *Black Women & Self Care,* this piece proved difficult to write because it centered around her personal story. Naomi is committed to making art focused on African diasporic herstory, perceptions of Blackness, community, mental health, and the Black experience. Her work is an important read for everyone — no matter their gender, orientation or race.

My Left Fist

by Naomi Moyer

It took another person to point out my pain before I could identify it myself. I was probably 14 or 15 years old when a high school friend commented on my left hand. "It looks like a claw," she joked. I looked down at my left hand, my fingers unevenly curled towards my palm. In that awkward teenage moment, I didn't give it much thought. It wasn't until many years later when I began speaking with a therapist, who included bodywork into her feminist framework of healing, that I became aware of the extreme tension, stress, and pain that manifested itself within my grasp. When I revisited that early encounter, the tension became intensely magnified. I began to notice this claw every day, every moment. In my sleep, at work, social settings and intimate encounters, the claw would not go away. I found myself massaging it, stretching it out, soothing it with ice packs. This burdensome system of nursing my claw dragged on for years.

How long have I been holding tension in this hand and why has it taken me so many years to notice? I can look back on many childhood pictures and see my left hand, twisted into a claw-like shape. The rest of my body is serene and relaxed, yet my claw stands out, juxtaposed against my calm demeanor. So what is causing this tension in my body — specifically in my left hand? I do not remember being punished for using my left hand or any accidents or particular moments of abuse or bullying that would connect back to my hand. I also do not remember any jobs that would have caused direct, or long-term pain, specifically in my left hand. I hold tension in other places too: my mouth, my hips, my thighs, my shoulders, but the tension in my left hand supersedes them all.

While growing up, my household was not a safe place for my mother and therefore was an unsafe place for me. I grew up in a predominantly white, small town and my school and community did not feel much safer. I was bullied at school for looking different, acting different and thinking different. I was called stupid multiple times, either to my face or behind my back. People questioned if I was adopted and negatively pointed out how different I was. Folks insulted and questioned my hair along with other anti-Black, racist comments. I incessantly yearned to be white, to just be the same, to fit in within the white-settler, Canadian norm. Despite all of these personal attacks from peers, my household felt much more treacherous.

I didn't resemble anyone in my household. Being biracial, I had a semi-present white mother and a very absent Black father. My white mother, who did her best to raise me, was in an abusive relationship with a white person named Bill. Between Bill's quick temper (frequent outbursts of yelling, threats, physical violence) and my mom's submissiveness, there was no room for any kind of healthy discussion. There was no room for love, for growth, or for safety. Being in the household, which was clearly not my home — but his domain — was like watching for landmines. I had to be careful with each word or action to avoid any kind of explosive confrontation, which was followed by silence from my mom and myself. I had no clue what family really was or any understanding of what healthy relationships were for a large part of my youth and young adulthood.

Abuse isn't always easy to describe and there are many forms of abuse that aren't so evident. Bill not only had a suffocating temper but often made inappropriate sexual comments. I often felt objectified, from a very young age as a woman of colour. Out of fear and repulsion, I hesitated to communicate, my voice grew muffled and futile. All I knew was that if I kept quiet and out of the way, less harm would come my way, both for myself and my mom. Bill had jurisdiction over everything within the household, dictating any activity that he considered a liability. The house was not a home, but a dark, cold, filthy place where I felt suppressed. I remember being hungry a lot. I remember not being able to concentrate at school. My safe place was either my bedroom or, better yet, the bathroom which had a lock on the door. Within these safe spaces I could relax, imagine and lose touch with my painful reality. This disconnection enabled me to unknowingly tap into a meditative state. Daydreaming might have been the precursor to a sophisticated self care routine.

I now understand that mental, physical, and spiritual health are all connected. Not all pain manifests itself literally. I can be physically assaulted on one part of my body, but hold that pain elsewhere, too. Or someone can verbally insult my hair and I may become silent for a week.

What I do remember is the feeling of depression at a very young age, without really understanding what depression felt like or where I felt it. Depression surrounded and smothered me before I could even understand what it was. The feeling of not belonging, being the 'other', despising myself and questioning my identity. Feeling my mother's depression, feelings of fear. Living in a household with an abusive person who promoted patriarchal values. Witnessing my mother being threatened, abused and controlled. When combining my personal experiences with common experiences that many young women of colour face, it all adds up to one big traumatization. The distress and tension I experience in my left hand is a clear result of this. My left hand stored all the pain until it changed shape into a claw or a clenched fist. All of the emotional adversity and feelings of depression were stuck between my fingers and palm. My depression was a result of constant attacks, and my left claw was a result of all of the depression I was storing in my body.

When considering a topic like family health, it is often easier to speak about diseases that are medicalized and somewhat normalized, like Cancer or Diabetes. It is less easy to speak of sexual, physical or psychological violence, but these topics still make it into familial discussions, often times many years after an incident. Yet mental health is rarely brought up at all when it comes to family and health. There seems to be no acknowledgement of depression, anger, or other psychological diagnoses. Diseases that are directly linked to us physiologically are passed down either genetically or manifest within certain environments or lifestyles choices. Ultimately, we can inform ourselves about these illnesses and work on prevention. Similarly, with sexual violence within families, if the knowledge is shared, we can learn to prevent it from happening to others. Yet, if no one is mentioning mental health, or the links between trauma and mental health, then we are not learning ways to prevent it or prepare our families and communities to deal with these issues. How can we learn to prepare for and prevent the cycle of mental health?

I have now come to terms with the fact that mental health is very present, not just in our thoughts and behaviour, but it is very present in our bodies and in this case, my left hand. Depression and anger can be linked to ancestral memory, but can also be a result of something that has only happened in our lifetime of experiences. I know there are huge mental health issues on my paternal side of the family, especially with anger. I know I experienced first hand what depression looks like after witnessing my mom being depressed for years. Her reasons for depression are very different than mine, yet they are still linked. All of this can feel overwhelming and we can begin to look and feel like one big, gaping wound. To cope, my experiments with self care that are linked to daydreaming allowed me to detach from situations and people I didn't feel comfortable with. I disconnected from my body and coincidentally disconnected emotionally. This detachment from myself carried over into other aspects of my life, somehow displaying itself in my left hand. My claw was an act of defiance, it was all the ugly and hurtful things I experienced ingrained into one, tiny limb.

My alleged youthful, innocent face served as a distraction from my claw, which I believed I could easily hide. I was disengaged in many ways, from my feelings, from who I was, from peers, from family, from school, from my mind, from my pain and from my depression. The disconnection affected many friendships, my abilities in school and in my career, as I was somehow unable to differentiate who or what was a threat and who or what actually had good intentions. Daydreaming helped for a bit, but at a young age I began experimenting with alcohol and drugs, leading to many years of substance abuse. Luckily, I am sober today and was able to welcome a group of loving and supportive women of colour into my life in my late 20s. For once I felt safe and loved and I learned how to build a healthy community around me with people who soon became my chosen family.

I knew, after leaving the household I grew up in at a young age, that I did not want to end up like my mother. Instead, I wanted my personal freedom and to be safe. I wanted to travel, be educated, be creative, have a career and make sure that my partner in life was a loving, affectionate, healthy and intelligent person who would love me for me, unconditionally. I feel like I succeeded at most and am grateful for all of my opportunities, yet I was unable to avoid depression, which has ceaselessly adhered to the blueprint of my character.

My chosen family has allowed me to have candid conversations about depression, family trauma and isolation. These interactions were difficult and challenging, but necessary. We can relish in the fact that it is okay we make mistakes or hurt the ones we love because we can learn to forgive ourselves and one another, grow and move on. These kinds of relationships are integral for remaining grounded and at peace with our imperfections. When reading books written by Maya Angelou, bell hooks, Audre Lorde, Zora Neale Hurston, Alice Walker and Janet Mock we can feel their personal struggles within the stories they share. In turn, we can source out mentorship through their words and learn to come forward ourselves. Now, more than ever, Black women of all ages, abilities, identities, cultures, citizenship, faith and class are opening up about depression and mental health. Internationally, we are seeing a plethora of articles, blogs, social media posts, books, zines and visual art where Black women are sharing personal stories about their flaws and vulnerabilities. This has created an ongoing, universal dialogue that is motivating and quite revolutionary.

In my zine: *Black Women and Self Care: Thoughts on Mental Health, Healing and Oppression,* I speak about how depression drains energy, changes brain chemistry. Depression is a shapeshifter. I now understand that my hand is a part of that transformation. The good thing about shapeshifting is that there is this flexibility within mental, physical and spiritual health to bounce and shift back into who we want to be, or a healthier version of who we are. Instead of seeing my left hand as a claw, I am able to see it simply as my left hand — something that is a part of me. I learned to see my claw as a fist, standing in union with Black empowerment or ready to punch potential perils. My left hand has been the force that somehow was clinging with perseverance and conviction. My left hand was essentially holding on for dear life, it was fighting for my safety, it was fighting for connection. I learned how to love myself through my left hand. When I started paying attention to my left hand, I started paying more attention to me and the rest of my body. I started feeling more connected to myself, who I was and what was important to me. I started feeling more connected to others and learned how to build healthy relationships and a healthy lifestyle. My left hand, which is also my dominant hand, is now a positive tool that allows me to write, draw, build, create and grow. My left hand is an essential instrument in creating beauty around me, and hopefully enough to share with others.

There are moments when I look down and still see my hand as a claw, or feel it tense up. I still have to stretch it out, massage and tend to it. I notice what triggers my left hand to clamp up and respond by giving it the love that it needs. There isn't one simple answer as to why tension may manifest in my left hand. There are infinite reasons meaning that there will be an immeasurable number of solutions. I have learned to acknowledge my depression and my anger and to forgive those who have caused me pain as well as forgive myself for causing pain to others. I was able to sever unhealthy relationships and nurture healthy ones. I am letting go of the idea of being healed to learn how to embrace my journey into healing.

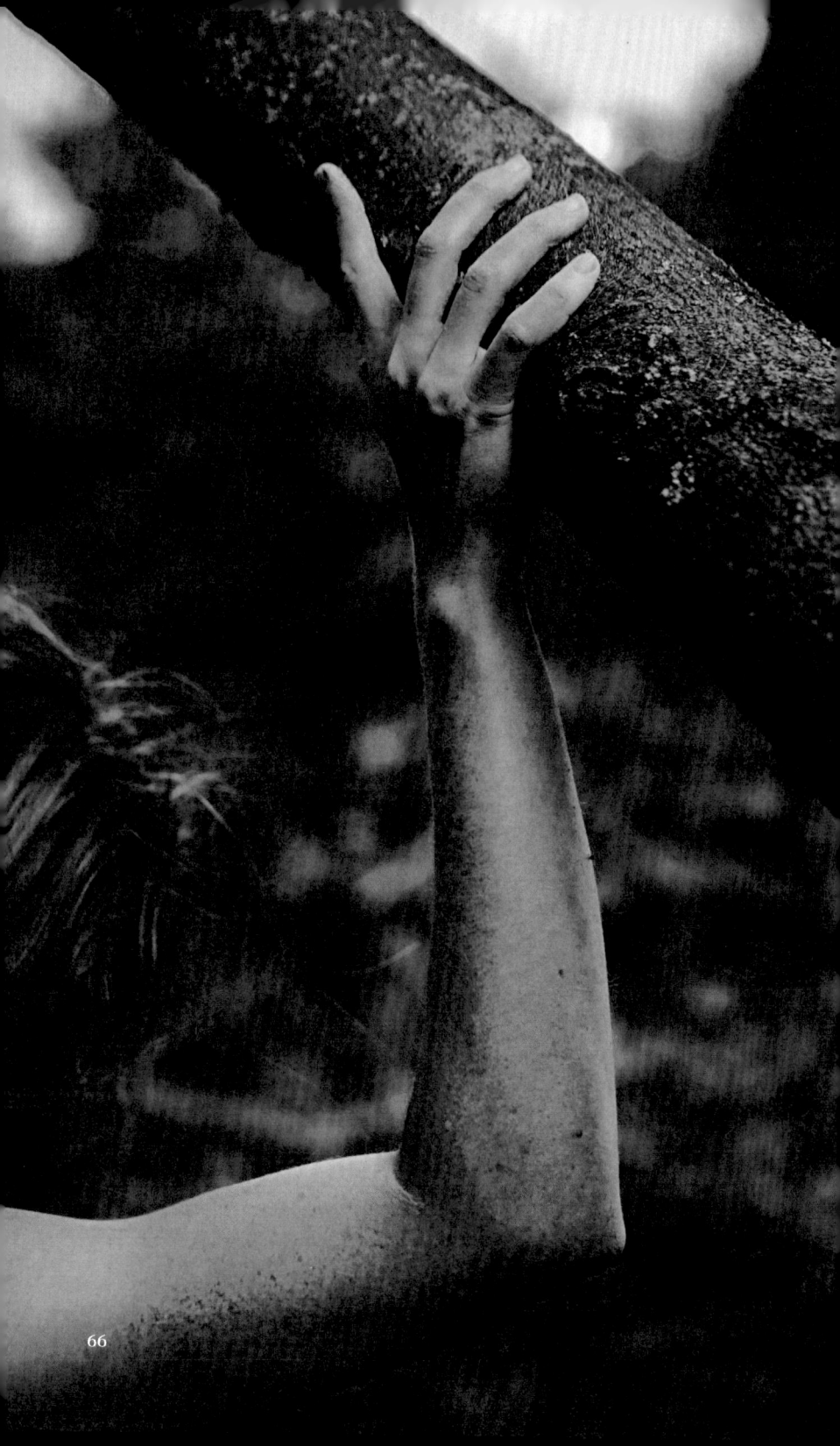

BROOKE MANNING

possesses a soft spirit. You can experience her quiet, unassuming brand of kindness in the songs she writes under the moniker LOOM, in every beautiful item she chooses for the shelves of her shop, Likely General, and through her work as contributor and co-editor for The 4 Poets. You can see it in her smile when she's hanging out in High Park with Jane, her dog. Brooke spends much of her time focused on promoting the work of other artists and is part of an important movement which provides a positive space for female artists to thrive. Her poem for this collection is both abstract and deeply emotional, touching on some very personal and painful events from her past that Brooke says she's been working on "putting to sleep."

If Death Then *Love*

If Thirty Then *Thirty-One*

by Brooke Manning

You weren't much older than a fruit fly when you
started to question reality.

You stared at your body
eating the cherry tomato ripening on your mother's
sill.

Someday, you'll be so full of you
so full of you
you are sick.

Someday
you will push your body
to grow so full of you

you'll be free.

In the first room you remember, there is a chair. On the chair sits a stuffed elephant named Effu. When you tire of staring at Effu, you cry to be carried into another room which contains a different chair. On it sits a stuffed man named Bob. When you are old enough to cry for Bob to be lifted not from the chair but from the ground, you understand that none of this is real.

In public, your quiet way of observation never draws attention. It is always your hair; It is always your freckles; It used to be your braces. During a production of *The Wizard of Oz,* you wish for Dorothy and you are granted Tinman. You, *and your imagination.* You, such an only child. You request a vacuum for your birthday — not because you particularly enjoy cleaning but because it concerns you that your mother does it so much. Your first pets — two goldfish — both of which you name Alligator. You understand that if one dies, there will still be another Alligator.

The doorbell rings. Your hand slips across the doorframe of your new bedroom, still unfamiliar. The ring your grandmother gave you catches and you are left dangling from your pinky. The ring works its way into your flesh. You are in pain. Now it is you that is crying to be answered. Quickly, your mother attends to the door first, and it is in those moments — the moments in which you are alone and in pain — that you remind yourself that none of this is real. Your mother returns quickly with your friend, manifested by the doorbell. He mocks your pain. You, *and your exaggeration*. You, *such an only child*. Later, long since freed and alone, you learn it is best to cry in silence.

Your mother cries in silence too. Her back turned, leaning on the refrigerator, it holds her. She folds a letter back into its envelope and places it on top of the refrigerator. When she is bathing, you push a chair as big as yourself into the kitchen of the two-bedroom apartment you recently moved into. Smoke curls each public hallway, imaginative stains on the carpet — *at least it isn't 180 Haig*. You scale the chair to scale the refrigerator. You find your name and mention this to her. It is your first letter. You put your only dress on, on account of the letter's request. Your dress is too nice and your mother makes you change into the purple sweater and brown pants she has laid out for you. You look like dirt, you feel like a root. You begin to wonder what the soil feels like for him. You wonder if he is a root now too. You hold your mother's hand as if you are the only soil to support her growth. You understand why you need to blend in, why you need to be her root. You are six and you are holding her, collecting her silent tears into the envelope you continue to hold when you are thirty.

You begin to dress in one colour, almost daily. You sit very still. Your colours bleed into walls, leaves, the lake, but mostly, dirt. At times, you resemble the dust jacket of a rare book. You get detention regularly for skipping recess to hide in the library. You wonder, what is the right age to discover Emily Brontë? You wonder if Emily Brontë is real. You begin to steal library books of poetry you still own when you are thirty.

You feel most at peace when no one is watching. You, *and your silence*. You, *such an only child*. It is assumed that your quietness is indifference. You quite like the assumption, especially while in school. Especially after you meet a boy who tells the world that the pain he caused you isn't real. You spend weeks, months, years, questioning the reality of the event. The world, like the boy, agrees. You tell yourself you should have known better. You tell yourself that death has prepared you for such loss. You convince yourself it is your fault. You convince yourself that none of this is real. Your mind sinks deeper into the soil that is your bed. You, *a dormant seed resting under a thick layer of dew*. You, *and your sweat-soaked sheets*.

The sun breaks and keeps on breaking.
You stare at your over-ripe body.
Carefully, you begin to uproot. You survive on the fruits of this labour in silent grace and when you are ready to share them, you do.
You meet someone that replenishes, too.
You are looking at and into the long lapses of time when your voice carries the quiet heaven of your individual depth.

To be silent and alone with you; You,
and your generous fruit-body.
You, *such an only child.*

You understand:
If death, then love.
If thirty, then thirty-one.

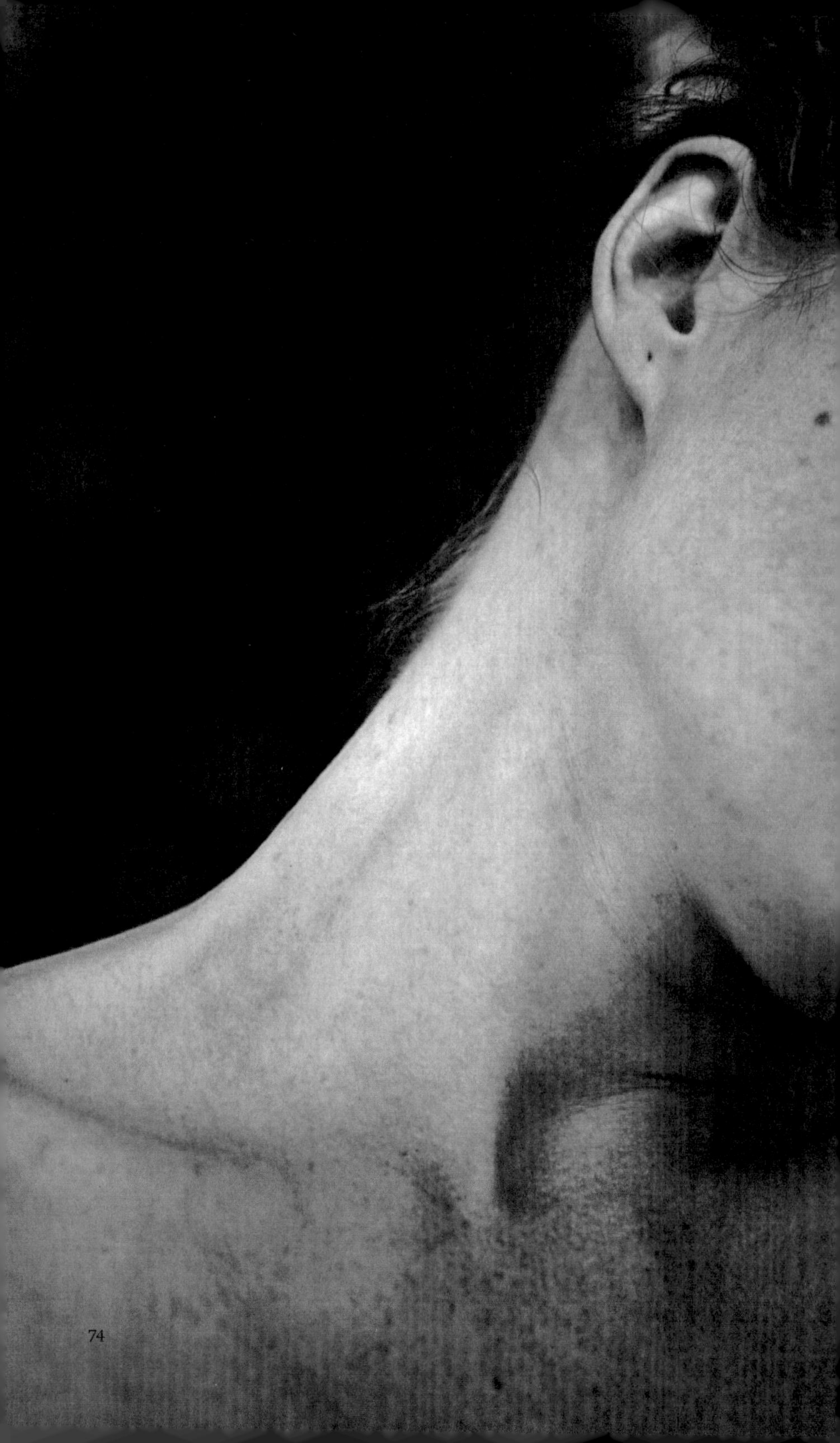

NADA ALIC

is someone you can tell your secrets to. She navigates the world like an explorer, searching to find only the most worthwhile songs to listen to, people to befriend, things to spend her time doing. As if she's ready for something very important to happen. If you hang around her long enough, she'll start to tell your secrets back to you, but in a way you've never heard them sound before. Nada has a keen sense of what people sound like on the inside. The quirky, somewhat surreal stories she writes for her zine, *Future You,* are not so different than the personal essay she's included here. Her work is almost always about the benefits of asking the right questions and then being open to answers you might not have expected.

#SoftasFuck
by Nada Alic

In the same way you're required to get vaccinated upon entering certain foreign countries, some kind of emotional vaccination should be administered upon arriving at the gates of LAX in order to prepare you for the social pageantry and the generalized anxiety that will almost certainly seep into your bloodstream when you become a part of the frayed tapestry that is Los Angeles.

I never took such precautionary measures before I wheeled my two suitcases into a one-bedroom Silverlake apartment two years ago, probably with Natasha Beddingfield's "Unwritten" playing in my head as I unpacked a collection of sweaters I brought but would never need. My therapist says I need to "stop generalizing about Los Angeles," but given that she spends more than half of our time talking about who matched with her on JDate that week, I take her advice as loosely as a post-meal mint that ends up at the bottom of my purse forever.

I was born as what is now medically referred to as a "sensitive girl" and I've since spent my entire life trying to calcify my own softness as a coping mechanism; manufacturing a version of myself that was strong, smart and most importantly: infinitely chill. But the spectrum of trauma, from the mundane to the catastrophic, is like stagnant pond water: It has nowhere to go and there is no way to out-chill it. The only way out of your own suffering is to let it course through your body like the flu, lest you become one of those people who cannot shake a cold for weeks. What is with those people? Gross.

Los Angeles is a "heavy curriculum" as my favorite spiritual teacher Ram Dass would say. And by that I mean, it is at once profound, depraved and more alive than any other city I have ever lived in. Not just because the endlessly looping freeway system resembles that of my own veins, making me believe we are all truly part of one celestial body and a metaphor that always makes me want to cry; but because I fell in love here.

Let me remind you that falling in love is not chill, it's not even kind of chill. Many people here believe it's a myth being perpetuated by our parents who live in places like Ohio or Dallas where traces of love can still be found in the peaceful bedrooms of some certain suburban dwellings. But fuck it, I did. I fell in love. I met someone and we did all the things people do when they are in love. We made out in his apartment complex pool, we developed a text language that only we understood, we borrowed each other's clothes and went to open houses pretending to be a married couple who fought over such things as carpet vs. hardwood. What we had felt real and perfect in only the way something that is not real and perfect could feel.

Not to gloss over the details but after nearly a year, it ended abruptly. As abruptly as when the moving walkway ends at the airport, except there was no auditory warning. As abruptly as when the heart stops during cardiac arrest. I was mostly blindsided by it. I don't want to spend too much time indulging in the details because, to be honest, it's still too painful to unpack. I was overcome with a kind of heaviness that had never existed within my realm of human experience, a fact that may say more about my naive, white, middle-class upbringing than it does anything else, but I was truly bludgeoned by this loss.

I entered what I felt to be a secret club of pain. Except it was not-so-secret, except every song that ever was and ever will be was about this specific kind of pain, but I had been too busy humming the melody, not paying attention to the content to notice it. I cowered at the thought of all of my previous encounters with heartbroken women and men as I realized they spoke a language I had not yet learned. But the last few months of my life was like a Rosetta Stone in the language no one in the history of love ever wanted to be fluent in.

Instead of hardening to it, I gave into it. I cried in tepid bathwater while watching late night television on my laptop. I wrote about it in secret Google Docs that my best friend knows to delete if I happen to suddenly die. I looked at my phone obsessively, refreshed my inbox constantly and checked my mailbox compulsively. I was waiting for something; an explanation or some kind of "JK, will you marry me?" stunt; something they'd one day play on the Ellen Show because of how fucking adorable it was.

None of that happened. Not because he was evil, or possibly a Lizard Person or some kind of prolonged hallucination I experienced after being out in the sun for too long. It was more likely because I projected something onto him which was not him, but some perfect version of him. He likely did the same to me, and you can only love a person's shadow for so long until the sun sets and then it's just you and another human person in the dark trying to find the exit.

One night, after a few months, I found myself lying on my back, staring at my ceiling fan in my one-bedroom apartment drinking rosé out of a mug, feeling almost peaceful. I stopped crying and I stopped feeling the tightness in my chest that WebMD told me was probably MS. I felt okay. It wasn't because I was particularly kind to myself, or because I owned more "Stress Relief" scented candles, but it was because I had friends that were there for me. It is because of these friends that I'm alive and breathing and MS-free (so far).

As I laid there, feeling the first tinge of okayness I had in months, I laughed with the kind of realization that you feel after finally getting a life-long inside joke. I spent so much time believing that softness was a close cousin to weakness and needed to be eradicated from my body. But softness, and by that I mean earnestness and vulnerability and kindness, was the only true antidote to suffering. And the only way to cultivate softness is to throw yourself into the fire of suffering and metabolize it; let it nourish you and others.

I thought of all of these women; women who came to my house and made me food and listened to my long-winded conspiracy theories of what my ex-boyfriend's Instagram captions meant, and sent me quotes from the internet and never once told me to shut the fuck up already — these women knew suffering. Suffering illuminated them with its petty cruelty, and they ate it and said, "Mmm, more, please. I can take it." They did not stifle it through drugs or vanity or status as so many people do. They felt it, let it break them, then as the body heals its own wounds, they rebuilt themselves.

I spent time with these women, these thoughtful, complicated women. Slowly, through osmosis or whatever alchemy aligns women's periods over time, I too became strong. I went from giving all of the fucks, to giving almost none of them. Like a massage, these women carefully undid all of my knots, even when they knew it'd hurt, because they had a clarity I hadn't earned yet, but soon would. I shudder to think of all of the many people who walk through this life so deeply alone, without the kind of cozy safety net of friendship I was lucky to find in these women. It gives me a greater empathy for the many manifestations of unhealed trauma — mental illness, violence and all of the neuroses that plague us every day. I truly believe we are living in a deficit of softness, and it is eroding our own humanness and (let's be real) letting the Lizard People win.

I fully recognize that we are living in a Post-Lena-Dunham society and that it has become v cool to talk about women supporting women. I had my own reservations while writing this that I would somehow perpetuate the commodification of feelings and add to the #FutureisFemale fatigue that is being felt across the internet. I don't know how to get around that; I don't even know where I stand with it. The only thing I know is that being a person is hard, so it's in all of our best interest to be soft. I happened to encounter softness in the women around me. Softness is not bound by ovaries, it's not even bound by human bodies. That does not mean that softness cannot exist in other forms: in your favorite record or linen sheets or inside a delicious sandwich. It can.

Regardless of whether I will find another man with a pool in his apartment complex, or whether he will like me or laugh at my jokes or tell me I look like a hot celebrity that I secretly also think I look like, or if we'll go on to create baby versions of ourselves that also resemble that hot celebrity; regardless of any of it: I will be fine. I know I will because I have the numbers of at least five women who will take me to Joshua Tree or start a podcast with me or discuss, with some degree of sincerity, that Tony Robbins is almost? kind of? attractive? if that's what I need. And for those reasons, I will forever pledge my allegiance to softness and vow to always be #SoftasFuck. ◖

ANGELA LEWIS

is looking for the moment when the right light connects with the perfect narrative. She's always wanted to shoot at her Nonno and Nonna's house for this reason, so when we first talked about self care and this book, she was inspired to document a very personal subject: her family.

This narrative starts with Angela's mom stuck in weekend traffic, on her way to visit her aging mother. Angela likes to picture her mom blasting top 40 on the car's radio, taking a final moment of simple joy that's all for herself, before her daughterly duties begin. Since the death of Angela's Nonno, Nonna is left alone in a big house she can't possibly care for on her own. She stubbornly resists growing old but expects her daughters to care for her as her health deteriorates.

This photo essay captures the complicated relationship between love and obligation. When should we sacrifice self care for the sake of a loved one who needs us? Angela asks this question with her lens and her heart, taking away the lessons she needs for a happier future with her mom.

ANGELA LEWIS / WEEKENDS

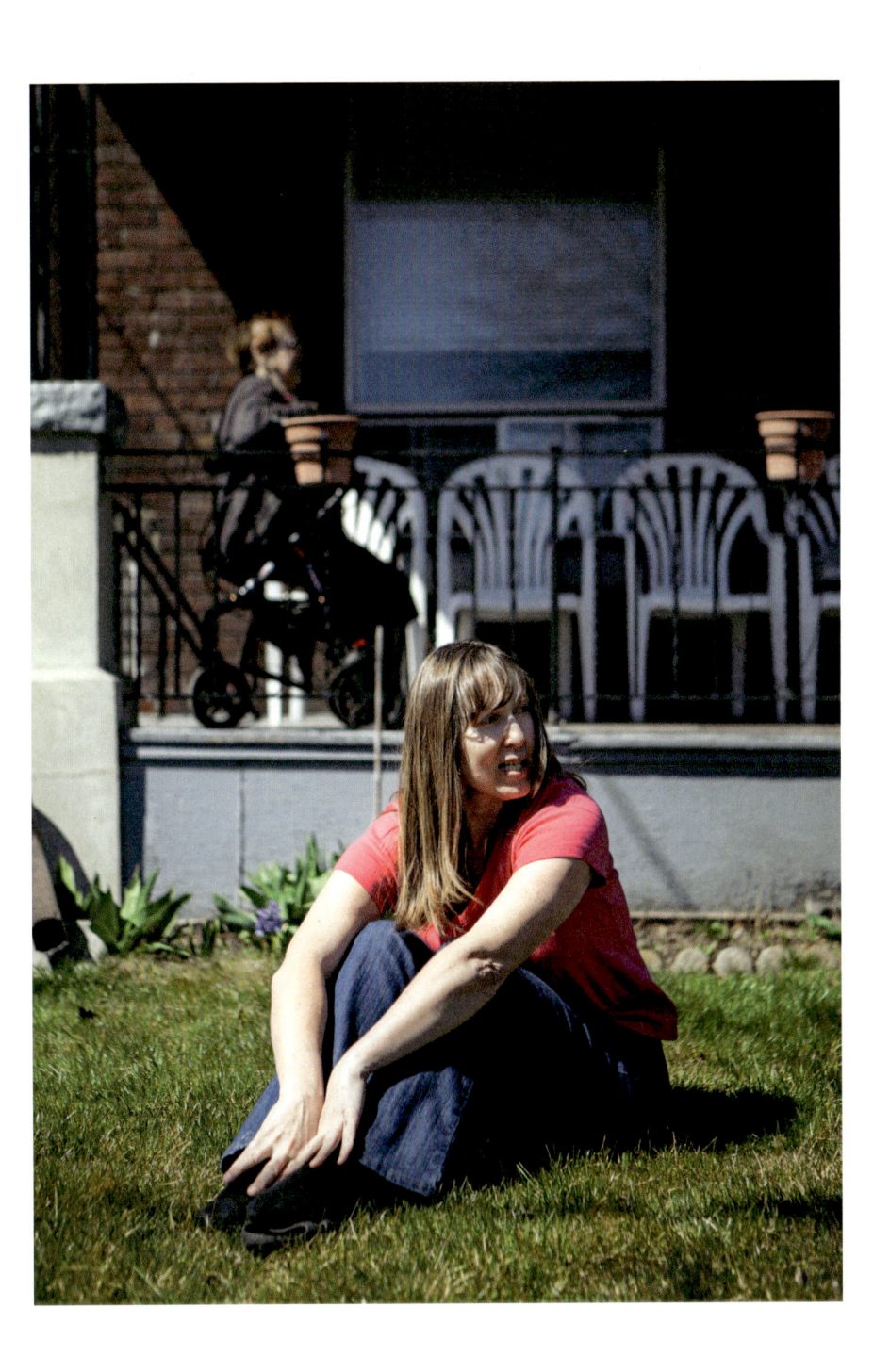

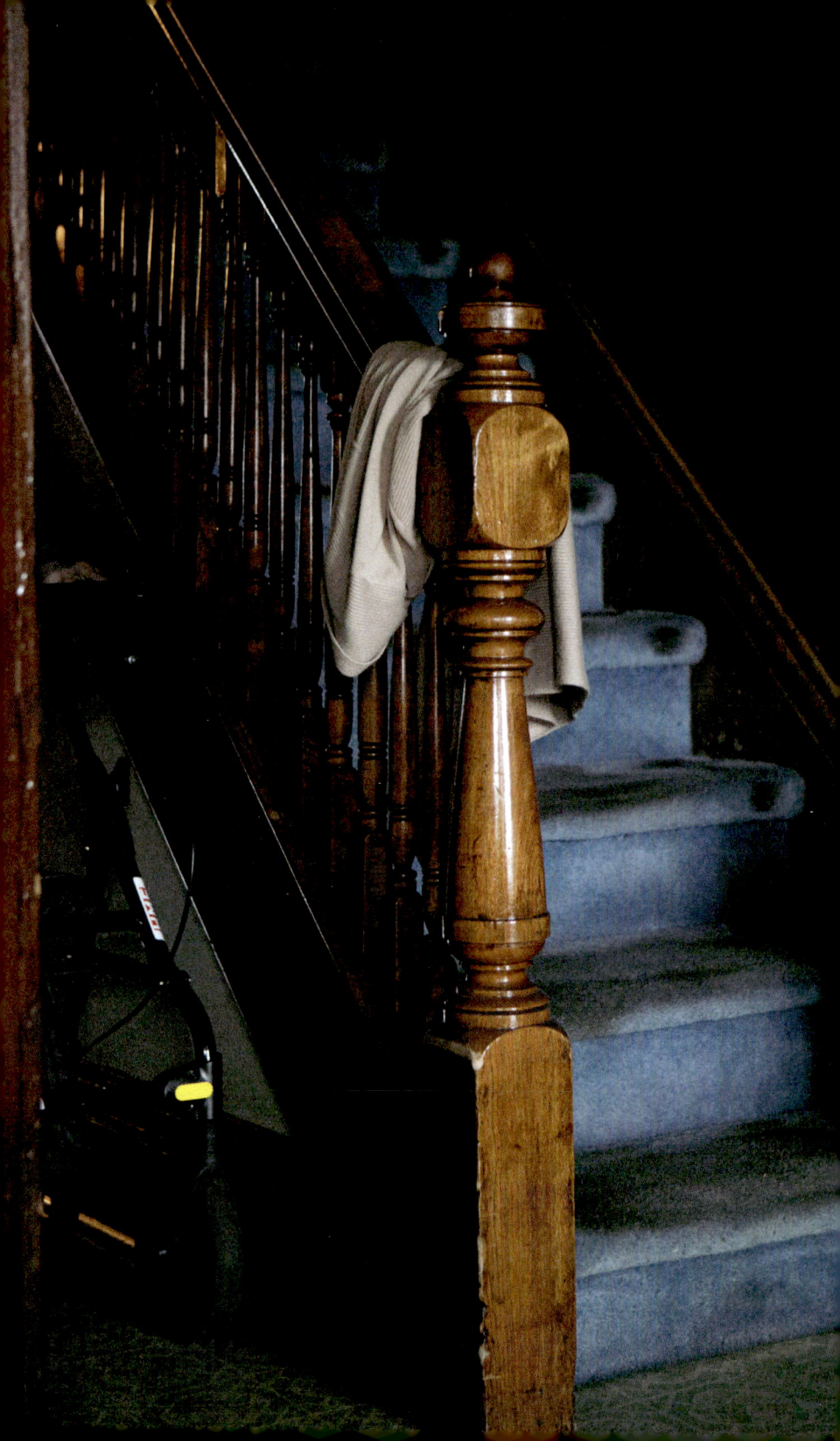

ANGELA LEWIS / WEEKENDS

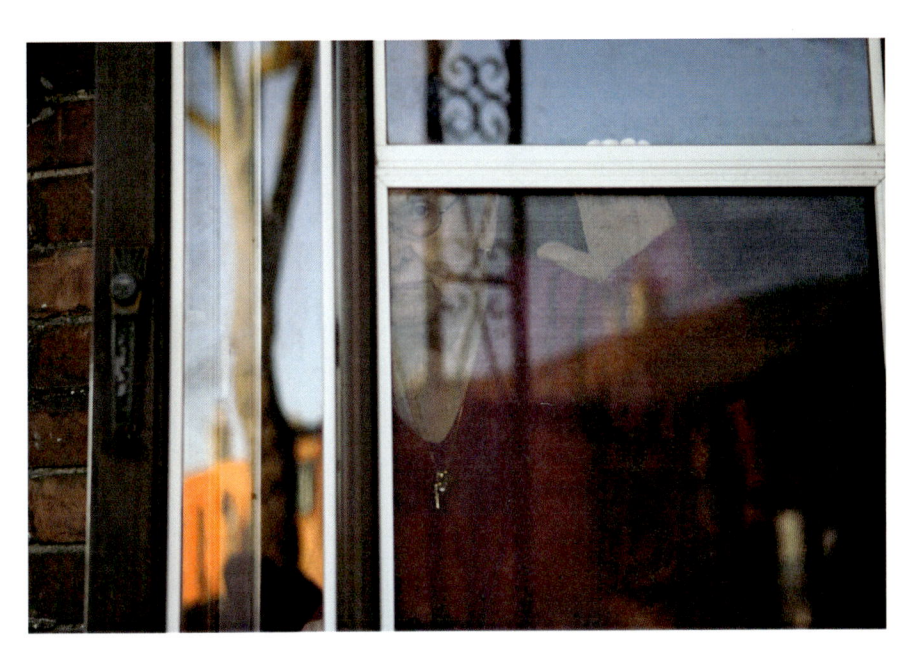

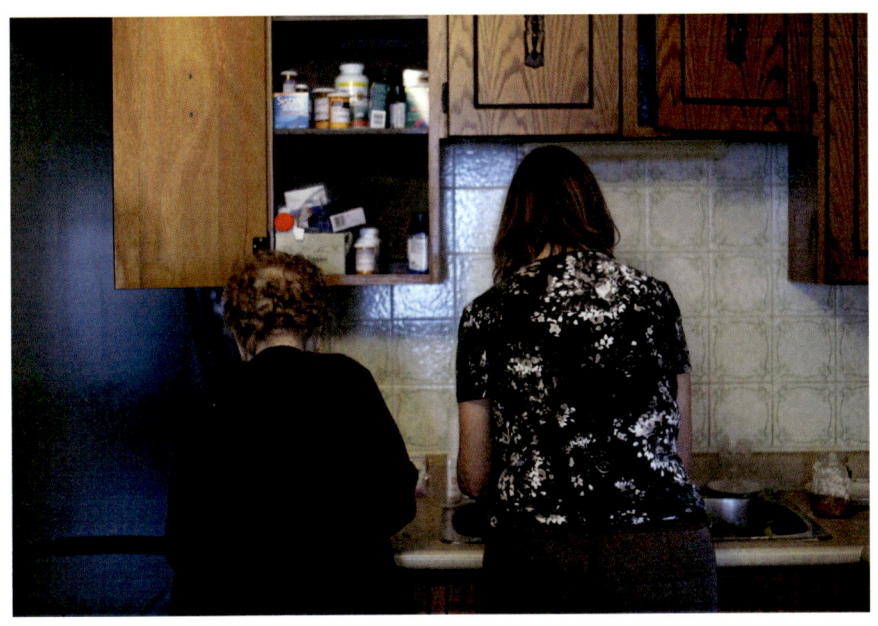

YOU CARE TOO MUCH

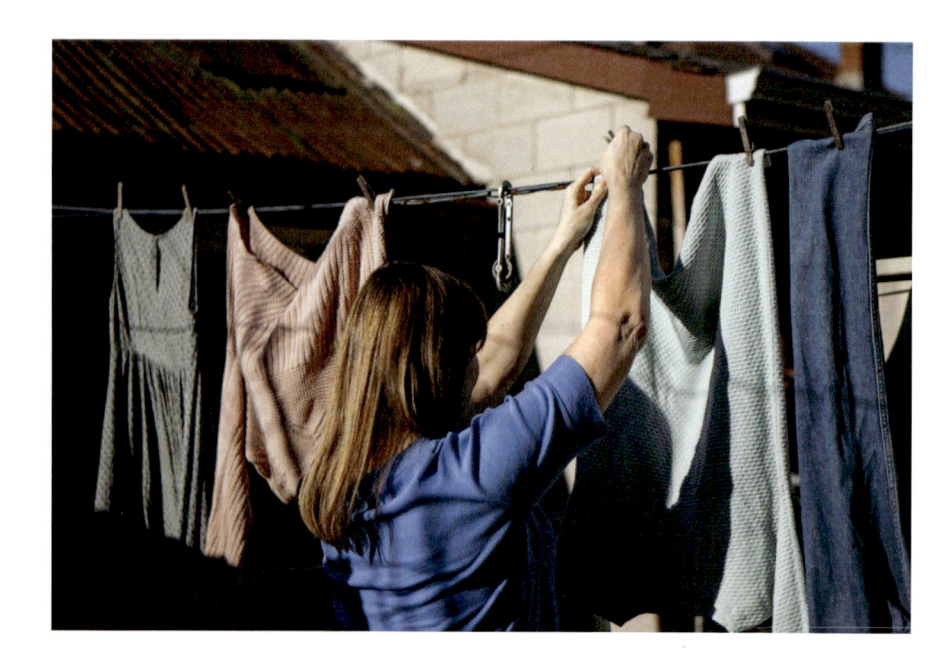

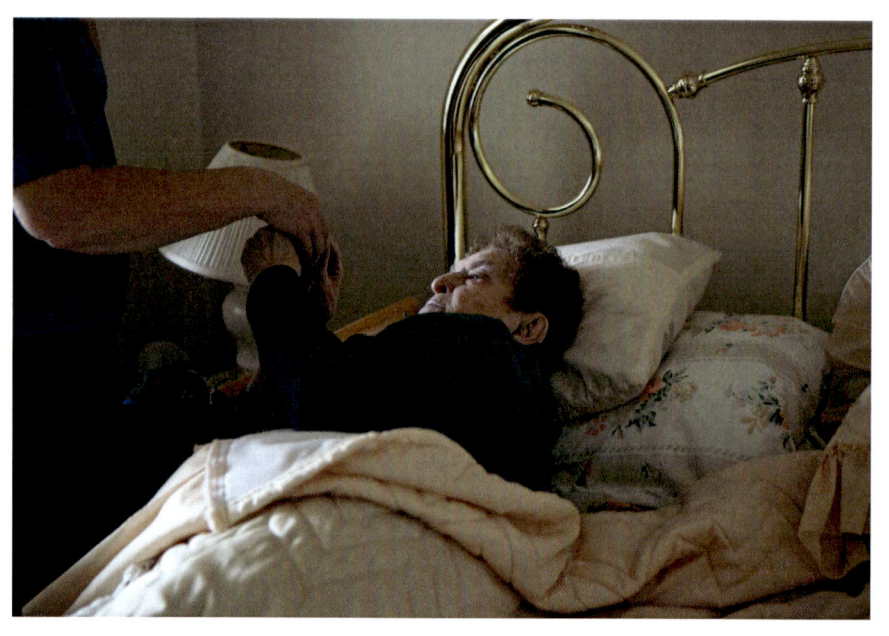

ANGELA LEWIS / WEEKENDS

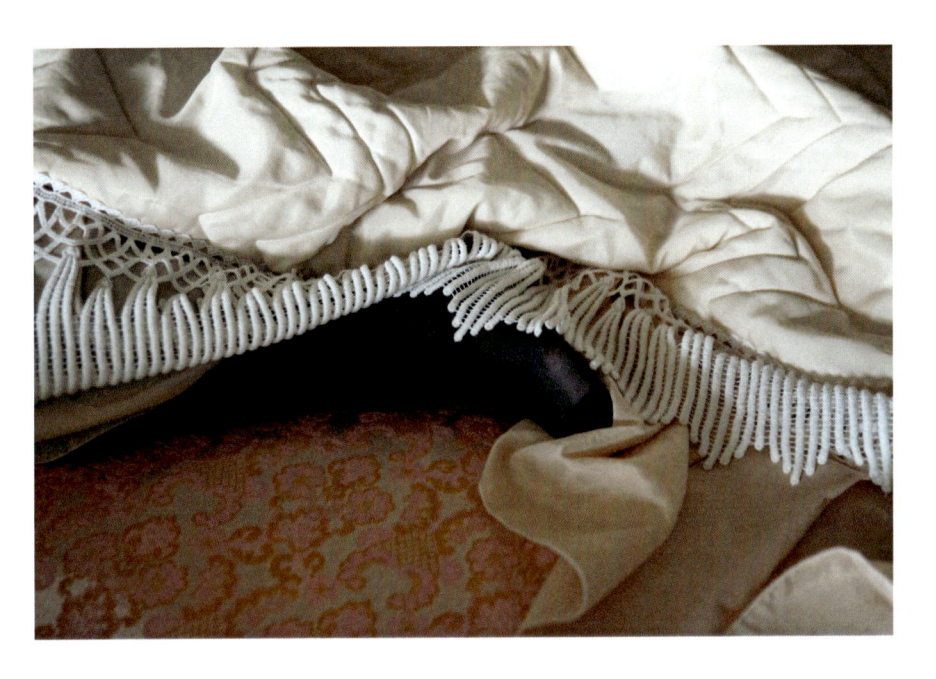

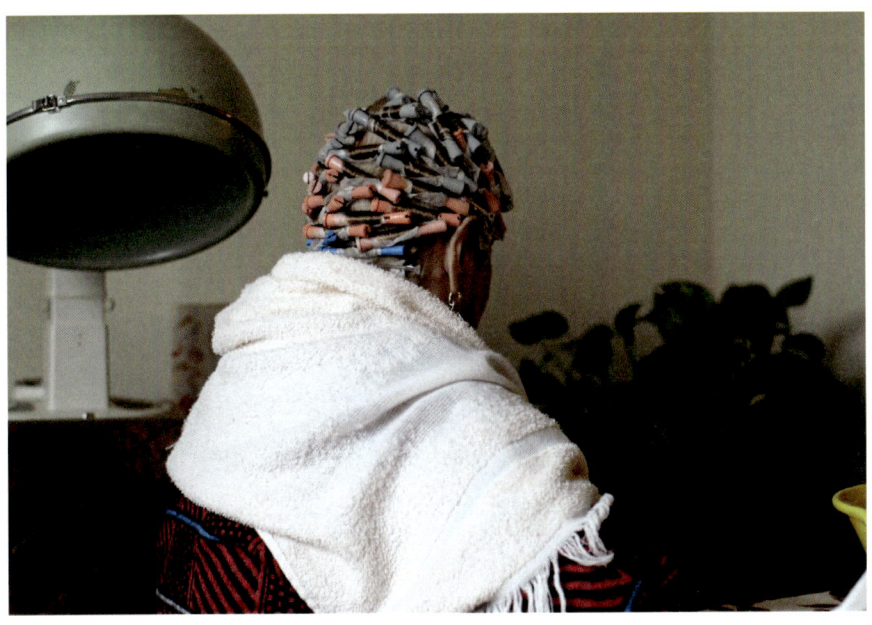

YOU CARE TOO MUCH

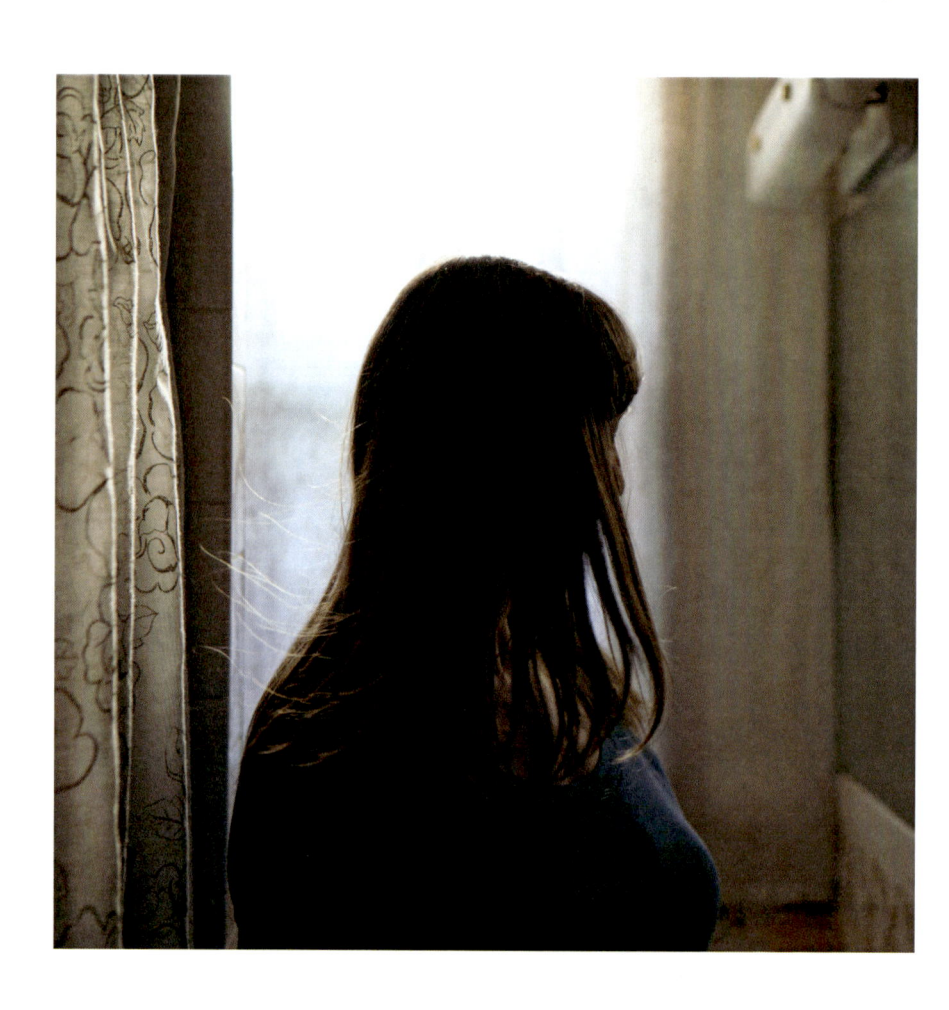

ANGELA LEWIS / WEEKENDS

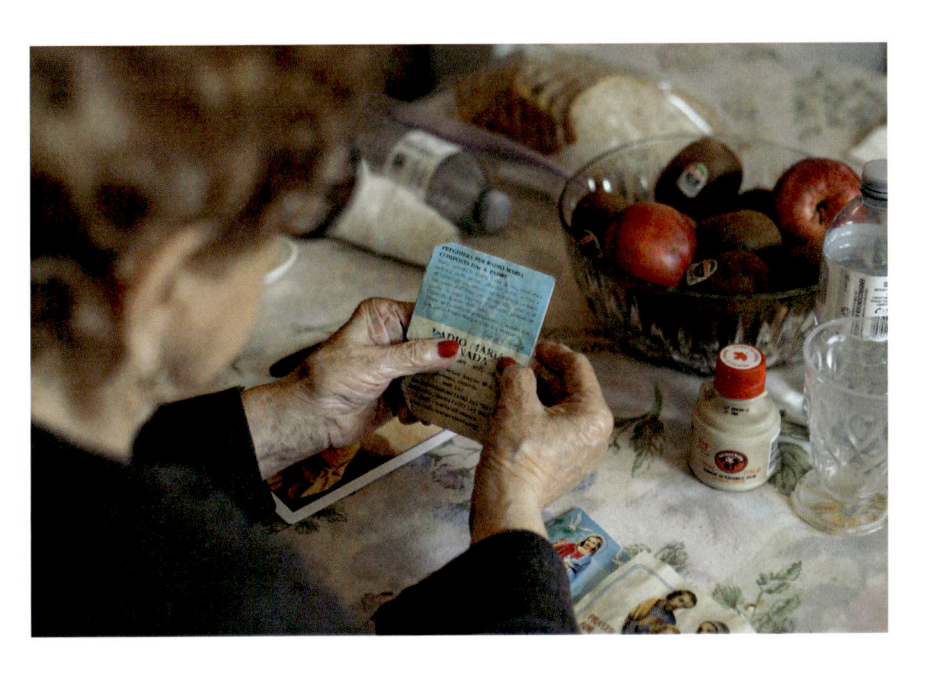

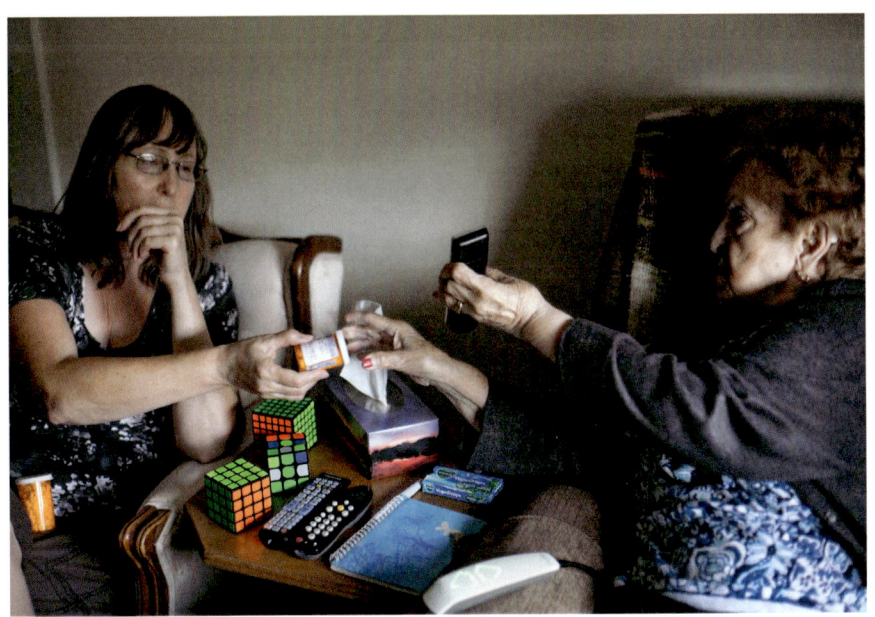

"TALLULAH FONTAINE

has always expressed herself through drawing. Self care became a more pressing topic for her last year after a breakup when her hair started falling out. In her early twenties, she didn't spend time worrying about her body or health beyond her appearance, but these difficult events forced her to take note of what was happening on the inside.

Her work for this collection is acutely autobiographical and centers around moments and feelings she associates with taking care of herself. The first image, aptly titled "Self Care" was originally created as part of a comic but ultimately stood better on its own. Here, she combines the stunning portrait with action-focused images — caring for her Philodendron plant and cleaning her apartment.

Tallulah currently lives in Toronto and is well known for her work with Purity Ring, including tour posters, merchandise and album covers. She is also the co-creator of *Home Zine,* a publication about the people, places, feelings and spaces that we call 'home,' featuring artwork by more than a dozen artists.

TALLULAH FONTAINE / SELF CARE AND HEALTH

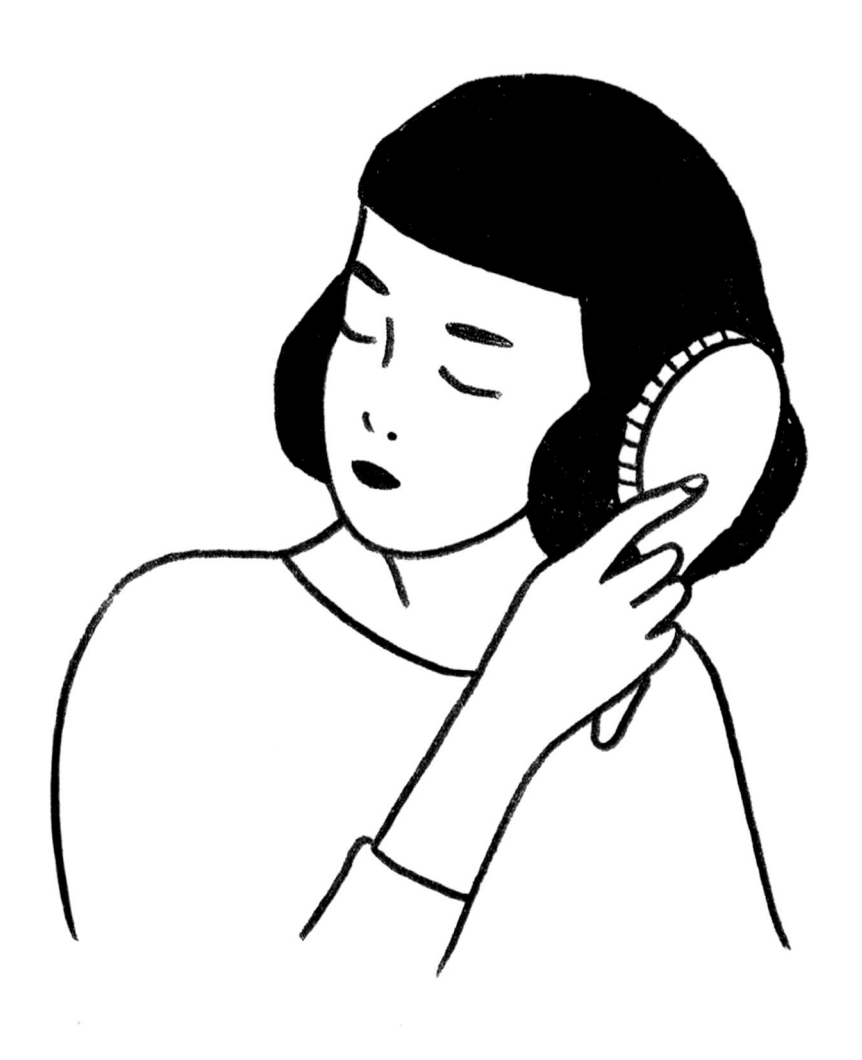

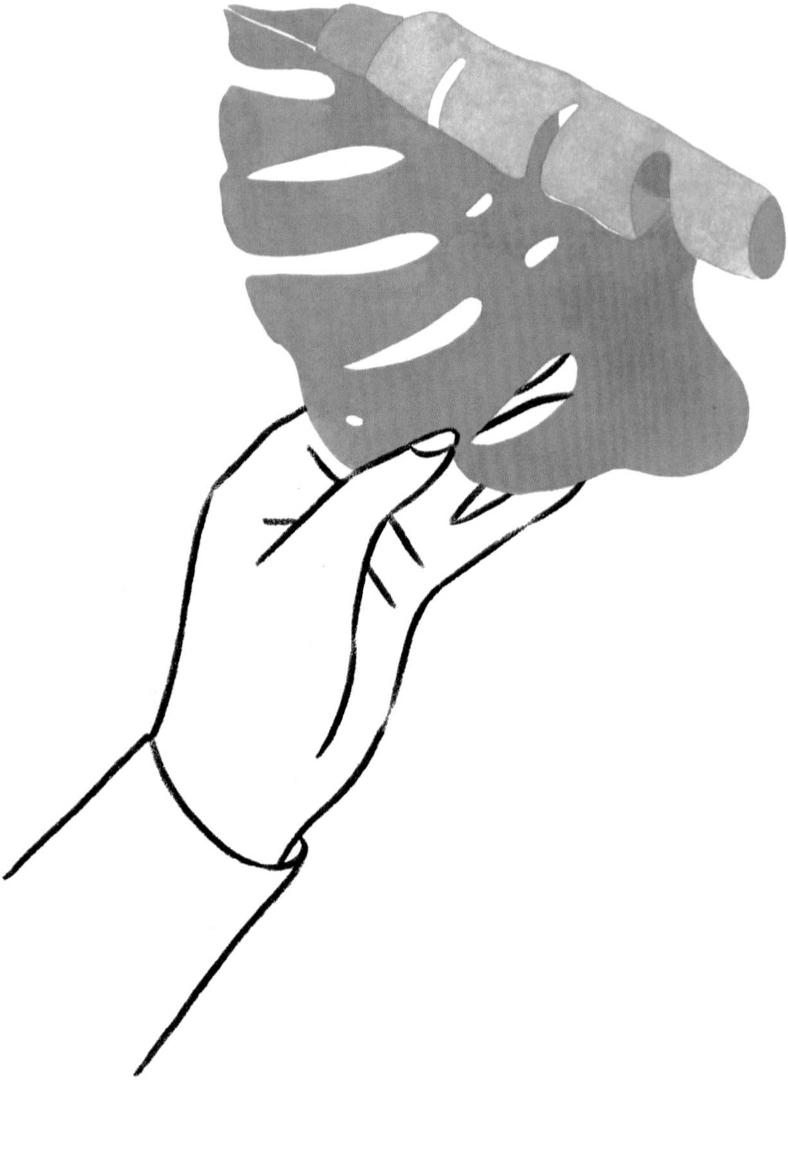

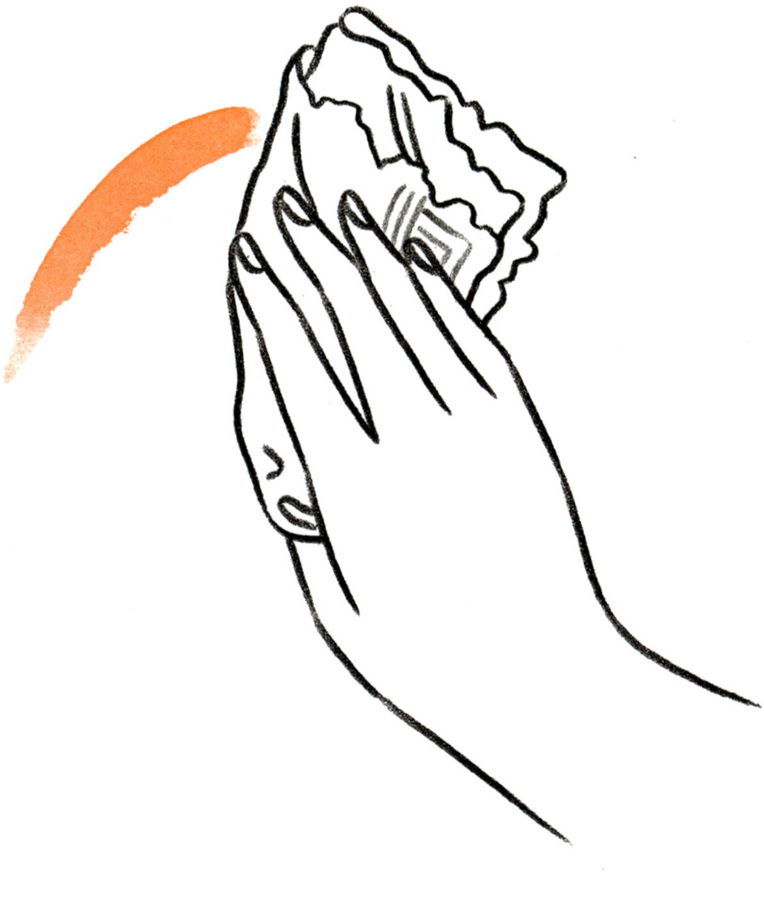

KATHRYN BONDY
wants everything to be beautiful. She also wants to know if she's the only one who breaks into **happy tears** at the sight of a beautiful floral arrangement. An artist all her life, the act of making things has been her anchor of light within darkness, and a compass which always leads her to a safe place.

    Kathryn most feels a sense of belonging and fulfillment when she's making work for others. Sometimes that leads her to set unrealistic expectations for herself about how much she should reasonably take on — mentally, physically, financially. Ironically, this project was no exception!

    Her ambitious living sculpture titled "How Can You Say No To That?" measures a dramatic 6 feet high, 8 feet wide, and 3 feet deep and speaks to her relationship to self care, which she says is "in a constant state of growth and decay." Like making art, caring for herself is an evolving process which requires maintenance — and sometimes it doesn't work right away. But that doesn't mean she won't keep trying.

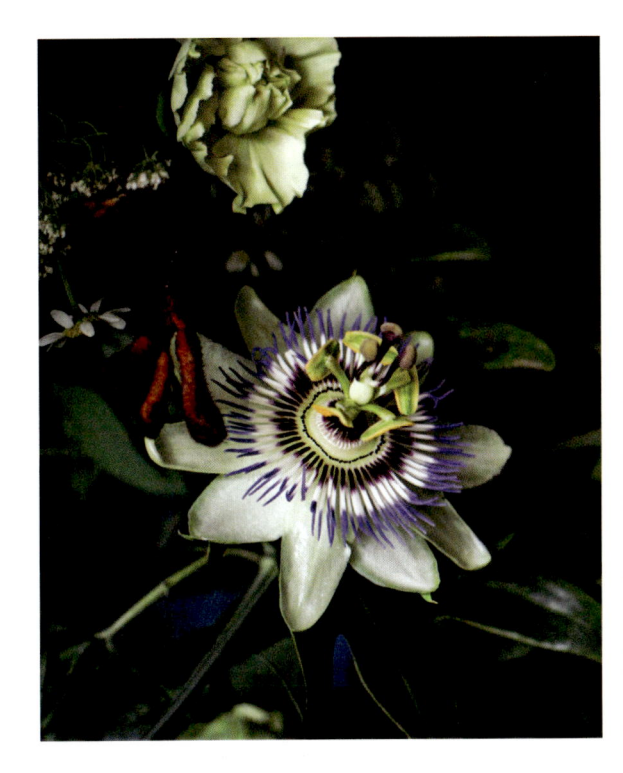

Exquisite details of Kathryn's still life, pictured in full on pages 94–95.

Materials include a hand painted canvas backdrop, bush ivy, lavender, chamomile, garden roses, carnations, Queen Anne's lace, passion flower, delphinium (and other flowers), the artist's favourite snacks and patience.

Still lifes photographed by Sara Keller.

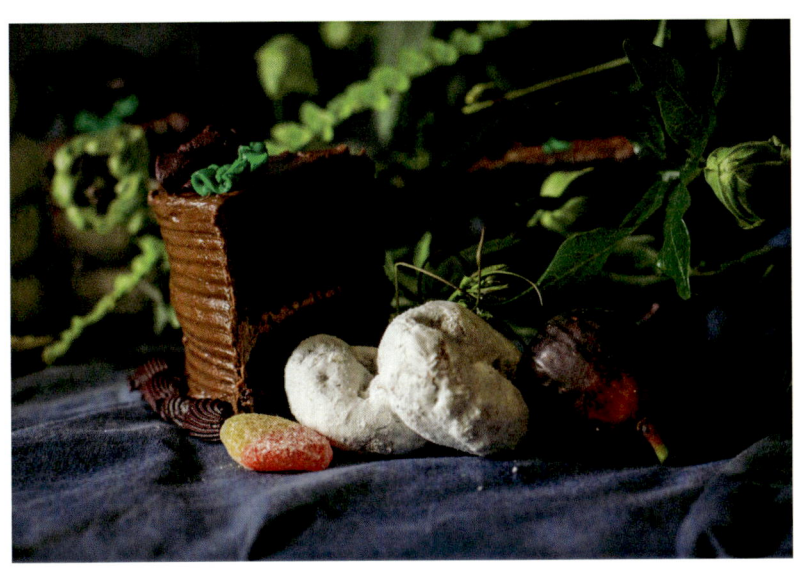

KATHRYN BONDY / HOW CAN YOU SAY NO TO THAT?

YOU CARE TOO MUCH

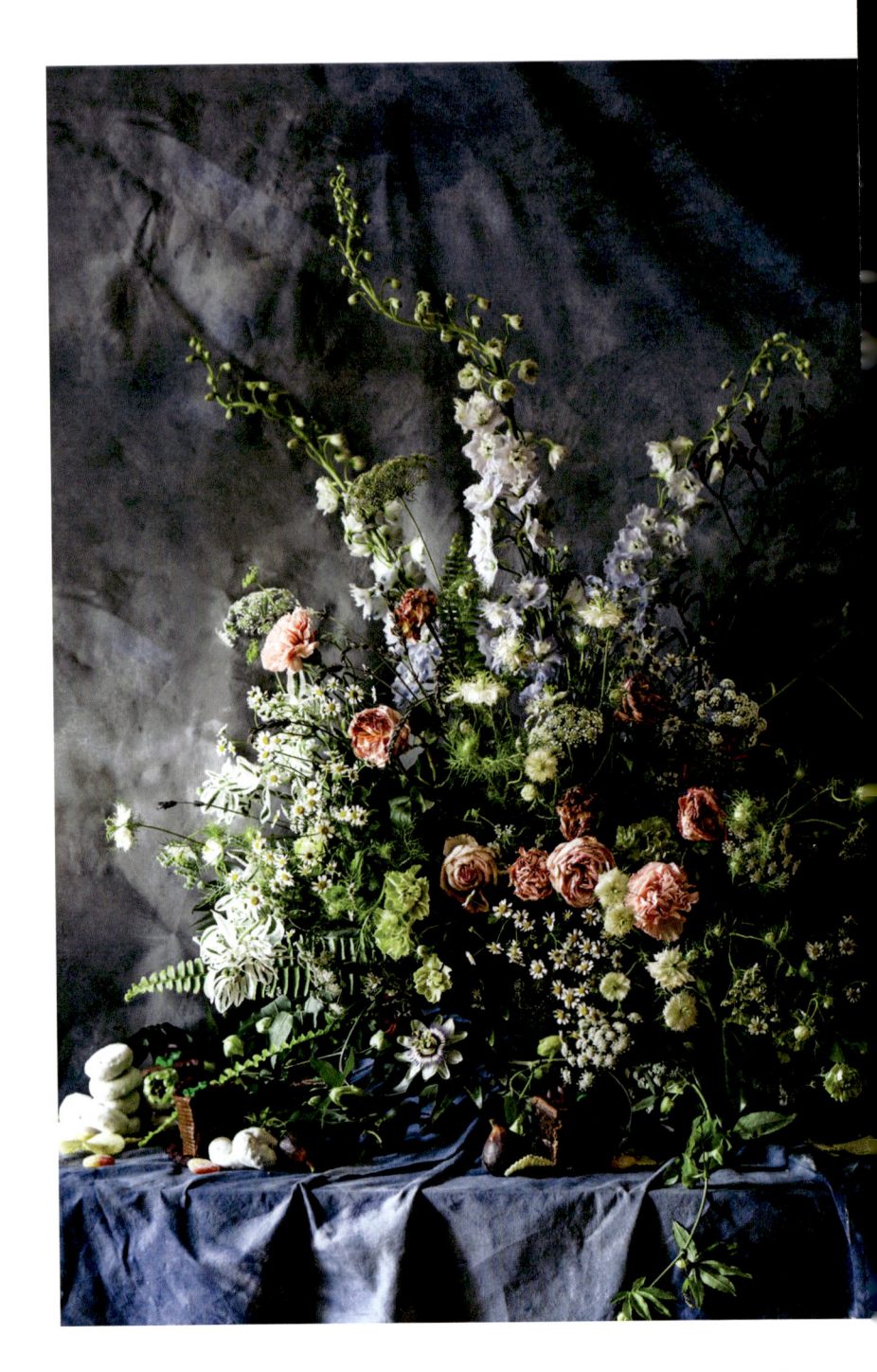

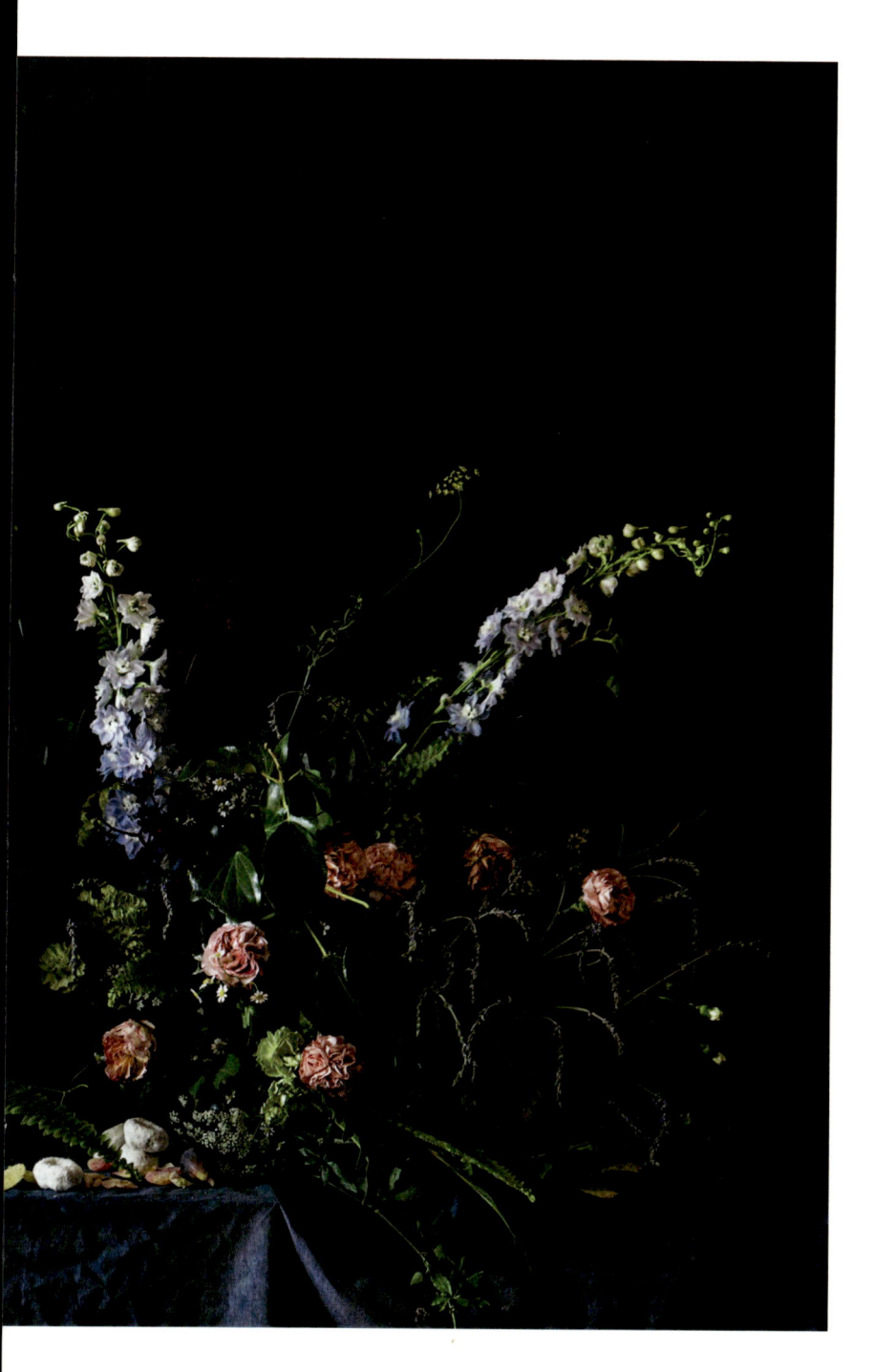

KATHRYN BONDY / HOW CAN YOU SAY NO TO THAT?
6′ HIGH, 8′ WIDE AND 3′ DEEP

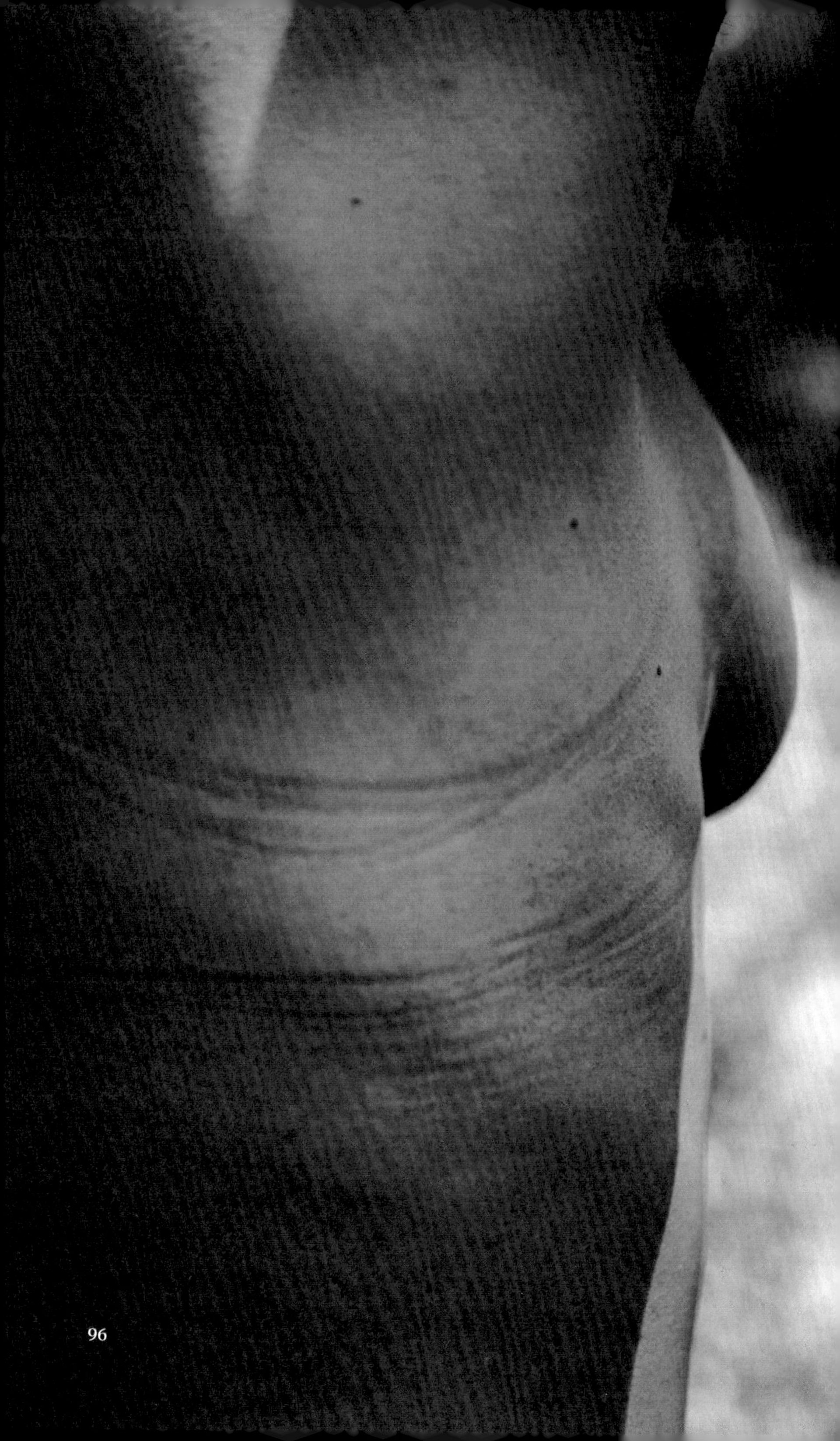

ERIN KLASSEN

was the first person to successfully travel through time—that's how I'd like my obituary to start.

If the human mind is already capable of bending the laws of space and time — think about memories, desires, flashbacks, premonitions and sheer instinct — why couldn't we also find a way to make time travel a tangible reality? In the meantime, writing fiction helps me connect the dots between learning from the past, coping in the present, and questioning the future. My venture as a publisher and editor through With/out Pretend helps me to do this too. By encouraging vibrant, intelligent women to make art, courageously, I am simultaneously seeking to understand: What is possible? And so far, it feels like the opportunities are infinite.

Becoming Carys

by Erin Klassen

> *One is not born, but rather becomes, a woman.*
> —Simone De Beauvoir

Every morning I wake up as a 52-year-old woman of Lebanese-Jewish lineage with dramatically large hips and a propensity for growing hair on her upper lip. This is the woman I've been becoming my whole life, until recently, when I started becoming Carys.

I'm usually in bed just about to fall asleep and then poof, I'm Carys—pronounced like "cares" but spelled with a "y" to encourage people to say, "What an interesting name," and to indicate I'm somewhat whimsical, despite my wholesome good looks.

The change happens shortly after nine p.m. I turn into a petite blonde girl-next-door type with perky triangle breasts and the most adorable button nose. If this new me becomes more permanent, I'll buy a whole closet full of vintage band t-shirts and mini skirts. That's what I'll wear day in and day out, with a touch of bronzer and dark burgundy cream lipstick to boot.

For 23 consecutive nights now I have fallen asleep as this girl, thinking about my future, thinking about my bad habits, thinking about the sexy bartender from Arlo's and what it'd be like to sit on his face.

Arlo's has been my watering hole for years, but it's not the kind of place where everybody knows your name. Jake, the sexy bartender, has been working there a year now and can barely remember my drink: "A dark and stormy, but not too stormy." They don't have frills like ginger beer at Arlo's, so Jake uses ginger ale. I thought it'd be a cute thing between us but he's not very good at flirting.

I work from home writing technical manuals for home electronics. I go to the bar to be around people, to be amongst strangers who, after years of seeing the same crowd, have become less strange than strangers.

I wonder if they notice me too, sitting at the bar across from Jake, making small talk with the regulars about the Blue Jays or the weather or the news. I arrive everyday around five o'clock and leave before everyone gets drunk, which is when I assume the real bonding happens. When strangers become acquaintances, when acquaintances become friends.

There are lots of regulars at Arlo's, mostly young white men who live near the bar. I see a few of them three or four times in a week, each time with a different girl. I ask Jake about it and he tells me about Tinder. "Oh, I've heard about it of course, but never tried it." Jake's lips tighten when I say that. He seems to be uncomfortable talking about any subject that is even peripherally related to sex. He's always watching his language around me, too. He warns the other guys at the bar to "cool it" if they start talking about women, telling overly enthusiastic stories about their bodies, or their willingness to perform certain sex acts.

I stay at Arlo's for a few of Jake's rum-gingers and am home in time to watch *True Crime* at eight. By 9:08 I'm in bed under the covers with the lights off, which is right around the time I become Carys.

———◆———

I started a strict face care regimen before I turned 30. The women at the Holt's make-up counters had helped me to graduate from "preventative" and "early signs of" labels to jars that read "anti" and "reversal."

My mother was really old by the time she was my age — most people thought she was my grandmother. She was too busy to take care of herself or worry about sex appeal. Busy working nights at the hospital, working in the garden, working on making lunches and dinners and freshly baked pies for my father until he left one day to live with the second family he'd been building in Florida for some time.

I've developed my morning routine for fear of a similar future. First, I brush my teeth and apply whitening strips to my lower and upper teeth. My face care products are lined up in the medicine cabinet with the labels facing out. Exfoliate, rinse. A thin cream mask to bring out the skin's natural buoyancy, and there's a touch of retinol to aid the process. Rinse. Cleanse with toner. Multi-vitamin serum for problem areas. Under eye cream to minimize puffiness. Daily moisturizer. Extra firming finishing cream to erase fine lines and brighten the skin.

My skin drinks in the lotion like it's been thirsty for days, like it's been waiting for this moisture it's whole existence, as if to warn me that without this regimen my face would immediately shrivel up to become the face God meant me to have.

I spend 32 minutes on my face while the whitening strips are doing their thing, then I tend to my "bad foot," which I've been trying to nurse back to normal for two decades.

The bottom of my left foot looks like World War III, even though my right foot has a perfectly ordinary sole. The professionals I've consulted believe it's a complex blend of stress-induced eczema, an aggressive strain of athlete's foot, and a type of psoriasis inherited from my mother's side.

My cobbled diagnosis comes from multiple dermatologists, naturopathic doctors, estheticians and even a metaphysical reiki practitioner who believes my bad foot is a sympathetic response to my unresolved feelings about men: "Do you get along with your father? Are your sexual partners satisfying your needs?"

> *My cobbled diagnosis comes from multiple dermatologists, naturopathic doctors, estheticians and even a metaphysical reiki practitioner who believes my bad foot is a sympathetic response to my unresolved feelings about men.*

I have spent nearly half my life searching for creams and treatments that will cure my foot but she says that until I get closure, and give into "long-repressed desires," I'll never be rid of it.

Sometimes I fantasize about calling the men I dated way back before I have memory of my affliction. If people could get a hold of past lovers about contracting STDs I could take the same approach with my bad foot.

"Hi Sam. I'm calling to tell you about some weird stuff I've got going on with my foot that may affect you too. I'm not sure if it's contagious, but it may be directly linked to the fact that you never once gave me an orgasm and were often unapologetically embarrassed by my 'out there' political views. I mean, these things happen. No one is to blame, and both of us are, for being self-absorbed and treating each other so poorly. We couldn't have known that there'd be permanent consequences to simply not giving a shit, but here I am all these years later, with one hell of a bad foot."

But I wasn't going to make that call. As my mother always said, nothing is accomplished from going backwards. My bad foot is a part of me now. I keep the redness and scales at bay by soaking it in a sea salt bath, then coating it with coconut oil. I never skip a day.

◆

My best friend Celeste and I have breakfast every morning at Fran's diner, next door to my apartment building. On my way to meet Celeste I almost always bump into my neighbour Edward and his dog, coming back from their daily walk.

I've never seen them leave the building but I hear Ed unlatch his front door across the hall from me somewhere in the same timeframe that I am making my second pot of coffee at 7:15. Because I don't see them leave, I have no idea how much time the dog actually spends walking and how much she spends being carried in Edward's arms like a baby. But whenever I see them arrive back from their "walk," sure enough Ed is cradling her, a fuzzy golden dog no bigger than a kitten, in his thin, tanned old man arms.

Edward has lived in this building a lot longer than I have, he and his wife were here in the early 80s before the big reno. She died last year, from ovarian cancer, but I rarely saw them together anyway. As far as I could tell, Edward liked two things: walking his tiny dog, and watching old movies at the local rep cinema.

He always makes eye contact and smiles when he sees me. I'm a familiar face, we have our little exchange down to a science.

"Hello Edward. How's Bogart? Nice day for a walk?" I fight the urge to pet his dog because people who pet other people's dogs and babies are the worst kinds of humans. People like Ed do the hard parts, feeding and caring for their dogs and babies, and we swoop in to reap the benefits of a quick squeeze, pat or kiss. This quick fix of joy is not meant for us, the casual lobby acquaintances. It's reserved for the people who have done the work. There's only so much joy a living organism has to give.

Celeste is waiting for me at our regular table. She drives all the way into the city to meet me for breakfast on weekdays. We've only missed a few days since we became friends fourteen years ago. While she's in town she can do pick-ups and drop-offs for her handmade soap business which she runs out of her basement. Most people would be surprised to learn how much money she makes, but she started the business long before it was trendy to use all-natural, organic body products, and she's built herself a little soap empire.

I decide to tell Celeste about Carys. Since the transformation has been happening for more than three weeks, I'm now convinced it's more permanent than a virus or a temporary psychotic break.

Celeste exhales loudly and rolls her eyes, like I've said something to annoy her.

"This isn't a Kafka play, Maryanne. It's breakfast. I think you're losing it." There's more spite in her voice than I had expected. Celeste is the most politically left and tolerant person I know. She's always been the whimsical one.

When she turned 30 she broke up with her generally tolerable live-in boyfriend and moved to Seoul to teach English to Korean children. She lived there for three years and when she came back she was tan and fluent in Korean. She also became a lesbian around that time, but I'm not sure if it had to do with something that had happened in Korea or if it was just coincidental timing. In all the years we've been friends I've never met her girlfriend, but she comes up in conversation: "Jan hates bolognese sauce," or "We just booked our trip to Knoxville—Dollyworld is on Jan's bucket list."

I wish I could be more like Celeste, and I especially wonder about the lesbian thing all the time. I think it'd be much easier to go that way, now that my life is sort of ticking along, with a steady rhythm. It'd be nice to have someone to share the grocery bill and watch crime dramas with again. I was engaged to a man, once. Near the end, we didn't hate one another or even exchange ill words; we just sort of passed by each other so many times that our apartment felt like a bus depot. During that time my mother was dying, and I was preoccupied with a strange kind of foreboding grief, the kind that gently prepares your mind for what's to come instead the kind that seizes your body like a stroke. She could go any day now, the doctors said, so I was back and forth to her house every weekend sifting through old boxes of photographs and financial documents, gingerly packing her

Royal Doulton figurines in bubble wrap. I barely took notice of the break up — I was focused on my mom. It wasn't until my 33rd birthday, when I heard that he was getting married, that I got blackout drunk and had sex in a nightclub washroom with a scary guy who, as I reflected much later, might have been homeless.

The conversation about Carys isn't going like I'd hoped, so I change the subject.

"I think I'll try the Muesli bowl today."

Now Celeste looks like she's seen a ghost.

"Maryanne, you've never ordered anything but blueberry pancakes in the fourteen years we've been coming here."

"I know. But today I want to try the Muesli bowl. Why not? Let's live a little! Plus, this morning I was reading an article on HuffPost about how flour can give you cancer."

"Ok, flour cannot give you cancer. That's ridiculous."

"Well it can give you 'thunder thighs' and that's almost as bad."

"What in the world has gotten into you?"

Celeste looks genuinely worried, so I order the blueberry pancakes with extra syrup and whipped cream. It seems to make her feel better, and besides, Maryanne's eating habits don't have any effect whatsoever on Carys' tight little body.

◆

I skip the last half of *True Crime* in favour of a little me time. It's 8:37 and I sit on the edge of my bed, straddling the corner to produce a sufficient amount of friction to get the job done. My go-to imagery is always a variation of the same scene. I'm at the bar after closing and Jake pours us both a shot. I look up at him from my bar stool, eyes wide as if to ask, "For me?" He purses his lips ever so slightly and raises his shot glass to cheers. From there it's just a stroboscopic picture show: Up against the walk-in freezer, lying on top of the tiled bar, sitting in the office wheely chair where Jake settles the books.

By the time I get off I've transformed into Carys and I decide to head to the bar. On my walk over, I visualize what it will be like when I see Jake and introduce myself for the first time.

"My name is Carys. I am the woman you have been dreaming about.

The mother you need to tuck you in at night. The daughter with the glow of untouched purity. I am the whore in waiting, waiting to do all the things you think only whores do."

The bar looks very different after dark, and is lit only by dollar store Christmas lights I have never noticed before, strung up in garland-like rows along the ceiling. Jake isn't behind the bar; in his place is a thin girl with huge breasts and tattoos across her chest. She's pouring a lager with one hand and reaching for a coaster with the other.

"Where's Jake?" I blurt out.

She looks annoyed, as if she has been asked this same question a thousand times. "He's off tonight, sweetie."

I don't remember the last time Maryanne was referred to in such diminutive terms. When she was much younger, her large hips and broad chest had inspired a certain gruff construction worker type to call her "honey" or "baby," but she had certainly never been the "sweetie" Carys is.

There is a man leaning on the bar and he is staring at me — at Carys. To impress him, I order a whiskey, neat, like I'm Clint Eastwood about to go to a gunfight, using my fingers to indicate my desire for a strong pour.

"You can put that one on me, and I'll have one of the same," the man says, which receives a quick but neutral nod from the thin, tattooed girl.

"Thank you!" I say a little too loudly, because I'm only a few inches from his chiseled face, which smells like a blend of fresh herbs and aftershave.

I collect as much information as I can through the noise. His name is Malcolm, his parents are from Trinidad but he was born in Montreal, and "actually," he just moved into the apartment building next door. I tell him that I live "in the one across the street" and this is a coincidence we both find hilarious and awe-inspiring now that the bourbon has hit our bloodstreams.

"Do you want to get out of here?" he says before I've finished my drink. "I have some vodka upstairs."

I hate vodka but I smile with my teeth to show him I'm easy to please. There's an unexpected lilt to the way I say: "That's a great idea," and then, because that doesn't seem like enough: "My name is Carys. It's spelled with a *y-s*."

Malcolm's apartment is terrible. The rooms are barren, decorated sparsely with Ikea art and furniture from the Brick. The jet-black entertainment system takes up a whole wall save for a paltry bookshelf which hosts two dozen books. From where I'm standing I scan a few titles:

Guitar Gods, How to Sell When Nobody's Buying and *Moby Dick*. He grabs the vodka from the freezer and pours me a drink. We keep the small talk to a minimum since I already know a bit about him and he doesn't seem too curious about Carys. I am outside my body, thinking about Jake while I wait for Malcolm to kiss me.

He gets to work right away. His tongue feels like a garden spade, chipping away at a gravel-lined flower box. His mouth opens wider than it needs to as if he's trying to fit my mouth inside of his. I've had too much vodka now, so I say, "Your mouth is so big." His response is to growl and pull my dress over my head.

"I'm going to ruin you for other men," is the last thing he says before we really get into it. The sex is hard and fast and uninspired. I half expect Carys' young, untouched clitoris to do the bulk of the work for us but it seems as clueless as Malcolm.

To keep from drying up I close my eyes and picture Jake's muscular, tattoo-covered arms hoisting Carys' delicate frame onto the bar, spreading her legs apart with the top of his head, nuzzling into her like a dog pushing his empty dinner bowl. While Malcolm is jackhammering, Jake is licking the spot just above Carys' left knee, and blowing softly on the wet spot until she shivers with anticipation.

> There is a man leaning on the bar and he is staring at me— at Carys. To impress him, I order a whiskey, neat, like I'm Clint Eastwood about to go to a gunfight, using my fingers to indicate my desire for a strong pour.

When it's over Malcolm brushes his teeth, brings Carys a glass of water, then rolls over and passes out. I don't want to fall asleep for fear I will change back while Malcolm's lying beside me. The shadows on the ceiling make comforting shapes. I listen as Malcolm's breath becomes heavy, a gentle snoring sound through his open mouth.

I fall into a dream that lasts for hours. I am on the coast, soaking my feet in the part of the ocean that meets the sand. I stand there, wading in the shoal until my fungus dissolves in the salty water and my soles become soft. The sun starts to feel hot on my back, so I wade in a bit further, but only as far as I can still see my feet below me, through the water. The dream becomes less fluid, and next thing I know I am sitting on the back of a great white whale, heading out to sea. My eyes are so open, seeing everything, looking ahead towards the pink and yellow horizon which is kissing the white caps of the waves as we glide through them, together. I am not afraid.

When I wake up, the early morning sun is poking through a slightly bent part of the venetian blinds. I've changed back. I slither out of bed so as not to wake Malcolm, find Carys' little blue dress from the floor to pull over my head and fly out of the apartment, clutching my shoes. The dress is too tight and too short on Maryanne's generous figure. Her thick thighs are shaking and smacking together as I run down the hall to catch the elevator.

Safe at home, I survey Maryanne's damaged body in the bathroom mirror. I massage a dime-sized amount of almond oil on my dry nipples. My vulva feels sunburned and my neck is raw, rashed. Somehow the discomfort has transferred over from Carys' youthful physique. The vodka is still evaporating from my pores. My brain feels like it's expanding like a sponge within the frame of my skull, a bone-cave that houses all of the scientific matter that makes me a person. At least, that's the way I used to think about people, that we are all far too sensitive, talking about our souls and hearts, when really we are just an accumulation of cells and rapidly firing synapses. My brain is set up to see the world a certain way, collect data and analyze it differently than the old man who bags my groceries, or the woman who calls from India to sell me life insurance. I used to think we were separate from each other, that we were destined for our own unique paths, that we were born with maps inside us telling us who to become. But now that I am becoming someone else, everything is different.

Breakfast with Celeste feels like a time kill while I'm waiting to become Carys. I sit across from my oldest friend, picking at blueberry pancakes, trying to think of something to talk about that doesn't involve my remarkable change.

The waitress who refills our coffee is pregnant. The two women who are sitting next to us are also pregnant, and are so close in size one might assume they scheduled their twinned-conceptions on a couples' getaway weekend last winter. Summertime in Toronto seemed overrun with beautiful pregnant women. A few weeks ago I saw a small-framed woman wearing a blush coloured pencil skirt throw up in the manicured shrubs outside the TD building. She looked almost regal doing it — her Coach purse in one arm, her other hand holding her perfectly coiffed hair behind her head. If the scene had been set to classical music it would have made a lovely short film.

Celeste became stiff around pregnant women. She lost a baby when she was younger, before she broke up with the nice boyfriend and moved to Korea. She said she miscarried at fourteen weeks and was depressed about it for a while but ultimately she was "glad that things worked out the way they did."

I want so badly for Celeste to understand that I am going through something similar — a significant life event where the universe is giving me a second chance to be someone new, now that I am old enough to know the things I didn't know before. I wanted to say, "You see, Celeste, I needed to become Maryanne first in order to become Carys. I spent all my time worrying about the future in an abstract way that didn't bring me permanence. She is all the things I have never been and all the things I should have been. She is born, unnaturally, of my own selfish desires. I am dismantled and she is my rebirth."

◆

Carys primps in anticipation of seeing Jake at the bar. She shaves her toned, bronze legs in the tub, ignoring the silky fluorescent scum lining the wall tiles that reach up to the ceiling. Her legs are my legs. I shave my underarms and bikini line too. My pubic hair is short and fluffy, so there's not much work to do. I scoop a mound of cocoa butter into my palm to coat all the parts of my body I can reach. I smell like sun and fresh linen and citrus fruit, all at once. Observing the significant gap between my slim upper thighs is mildly arousing. Again, I practice what I will say to Jake, when he takes me to the back room. "I am the vessel for your unborn children, I am your hopes and dreams personified, I am the precious thing that will save you from yourself."

In the lobby, I run into Edward, who is pacing around the retaining beam looking frantic. He is holding a stack of posters and wearing masking tape around his wrist like a bracelet. He is in despair.

"Hello there," I say gently so as not to startle him, as he appears to be in his own world. "Is something wrong?"

He does a double take when he looks at me in my electric blue get up. "My dog," his voice quivers. "My dog is gone. I can't find her. I've been looking all day and now it's dark and no one's called yet..." He gestures with the stack of posters which feature a photo of Bogart and type that reads "LOST!! Sandy coloured Norfolk Terrier. Answers to BOGART. $1000 reward. Please call Edward."

Poor Edward, I think. That dog is all he has.

"Someone will call, I'm sure she's okay. But it won't do you any good to give yourself a heart attack, will it?"

He looks at Carys the same way he looks at me when I'm Maryanne. With sincerity. His posture softens a bit, like he's releasing some of his anxiety and replacing it with positive thinking.

If I squint, Edward looks like an old punk rocker, like a very frail Thurston Moore or John Doe with less hair. His pants are cuffed and sit right at his ankles, his shirt is nicely fitted, and he's wearing brown Converse. Actually, Edward is kind of attractive.

The next moments are fueled purely by instinct. We exchange a few more pleasantries and I invite myself upstairs to Edward's place, to watch a movie. "It will take your mind off things while you're waiting for someone to call about finding your dog." I touch his arm and tilt my head.

> He looks at Carys the same way he looks at me when I'm Maryanne.

We're only halfway through a bottle of wine and 30 minutes into *Vertigo* before I pounce on Edward like a cat in heat. Oddly, he doesn't seem surprised. He makes space for me to sink into him, grabs my face with his hands while his mouth meets mine in practiced — but sensual — assent.

I barely even think about Jake. Edward's hands are all over me in all the right ways, eagerly exploring the parts that men usually leave behind, like

YOU CARE TOO MUCH

the curve of my waist and back of my thigh, right next to the crease of flesh that becomes my ass. My underwear is still caught around my calves when I slip onto him. He fits beautifully.

I can feel Edward's sperm passing through Carys' cervix, working like millions of white whales through the frothy caps of restless ocean waves. When it is over, Carys' body might be starting something new. An end is also a beginning.

Edward's heart is beating with vigor and his breaths are short and desperate. I lie on his body in child's pose, with my ear pressed up against his heart. I need to focus all of my listening skills to make sure his heart slows down, keeps beating. "Don't quit on me now Edward," I whisper, my hot breath on his ear lobe.

I can tell that he needs me in a way no one had needed me before. This fills me with comfort — and my mother's voice — that I will never really be anyone if I am not something crucial to someone else.

He's sleeping now. I think about our future together, about how people in shopping centers will think I'm his granddaughter, but that it won't bother us at all. One day, I'll tell him about how I became Carys and he'll understand completely and say, "I remember Maryanne. She was a nice woman." And we'll reminisce about the way she laughed with her whole body and the conversations they had about the nut jobs on the tenants' board.

I think about how Edward won't be around forever, and that soon Carys will be confronted by a deep, internal need to be needed. When that happens, she'll want to become someone else. Find a next shape to fit a new set of desires. It will start with a secret wish, a lover's gaze, a closet full of mini skirts.

It was almost morning, and I was learning — just in time — that the process of becoming someone was not as complicated as it had seemed the first time around. ▶

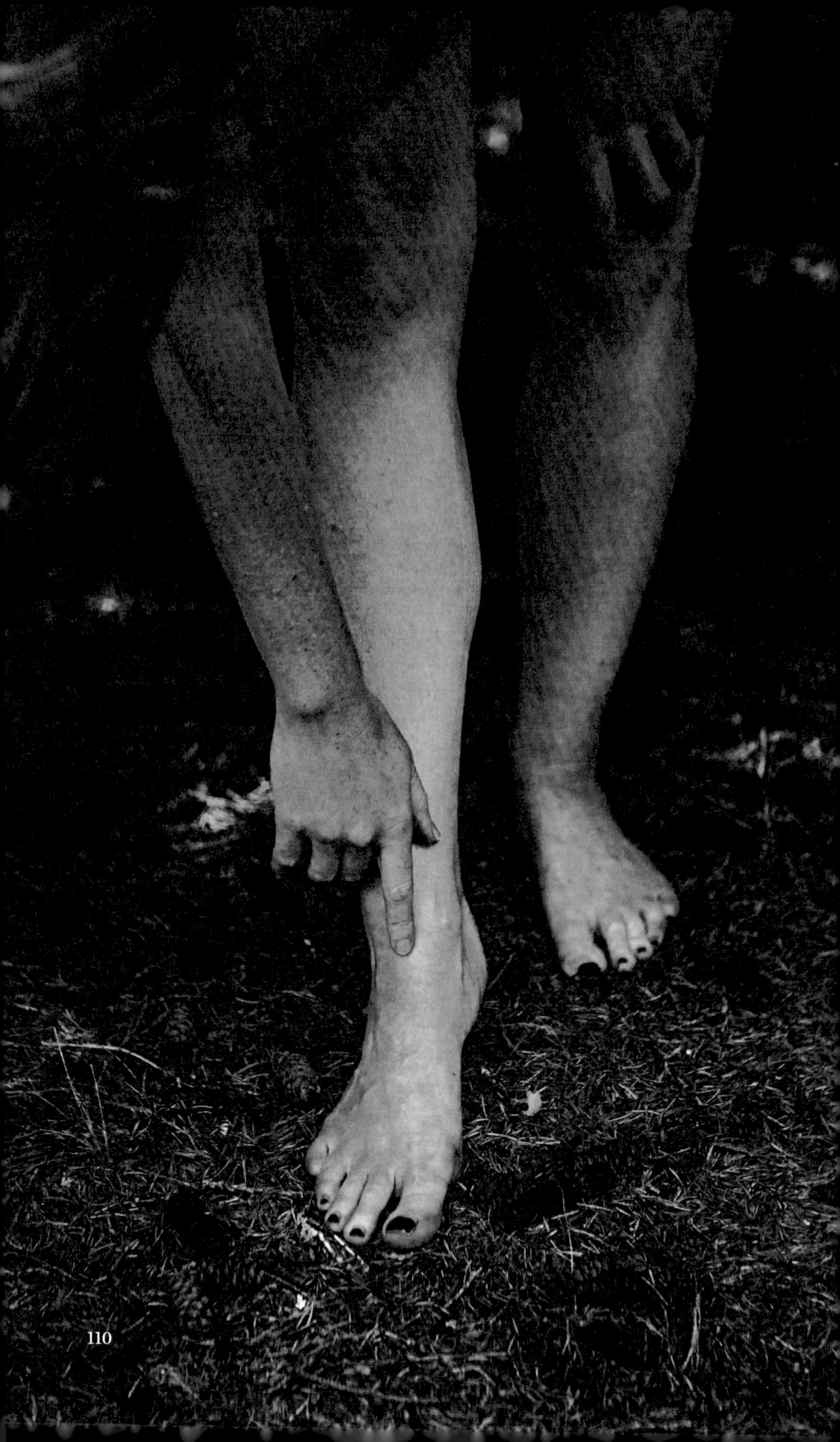

ADINA TARRALIK DUFFY

is deeply connected to the land she calls home, Coral Harbour, Nunavut. Designer, carver, writer and vinyl collector, Adina feels best when she's carving bone to create unique jewelry for her business, Ugly Fish. Her work is natural and from the earth, made from antlers, claws, hooves, beluga vertebrae and ivory that she and her fiancé gather from the land or receive as gifts from their friends, family and neighbours. Adina grew up very close to her maternal grandparents, who didn't speak English. As is visible in her work, Adina carries with her the love and wisdom of her grandparents, as well as the influence of the Nunavut community.

My Grandfather's House

by Adina Tarralik Duffy

The first time I walked through the door, after they had both passed, I didn't expect the heavy wave of grief to greet me so completely, engulfing all my senses. Mostly it was the smell. It was so thick. The scent of their lives still hung in the air as though you could reach out and touch them. If you kept your eyes closed you could almost believe they were still there. I stood in the porch unable to move. My eyes still closed, I held my hand over my mouth to keep the intense weeping sound from escaping my lips. Hot tears filled my eyes and dropped to the dusty plywood flooring. How can I do this? How can I live in this house? How can I call it my own when it's still so heavy with their memory?

Finally I composed myself and walked around the house, suddenly numb to any emotion, as though there was a fine layer of haze between myself and the reality around me. They are gone and I am here, in their house.

For the first year, I can't sleep in their room. My fiancé Aaron, my growing belly and I sleep in one of the spare rooms.

It has been 17 years since I moved away from this town. We decided to move back when we found out we were expecting. Between hugs, joyous tears, nervous bursts of laughter and staring off in a daze, we were unable to say much more than a few shock-infused sentences. My father had casually asked us over a year ago if we wanted to move up north to help with the family business, the hotel they've run since I was about six years old. Since then the idea had been stewing about in the back of our minds.

My grandparents' house had been vacant for some time and my mother had asked us if we wanted to live there. I wasn't entirely sure how I felt about it but the romance of home was calling and with the news of baby-on-the-way, we were finally ready to answer. We packed up our lives and headed to my hometown of about 800 people, located on Southampton Island, 290 kilometres below the Arctic Circle.

Somedays it feels like the only place on earth I can breathe properly. Somedays I can feel the claustrophobia caving in on me. The sprawling tundra that reaches for miles, the ocean that breaks and blends with the sky, the endless rock and gravel that covers this island like the face of some extraterrestrial landscape. The wide open spread of the land acutely contrasted against the intensely inescapable closeness of our community. There is no anonymity here. Living here can make you feel as far away as the moon or as close to your roots as if you were sleeping in your mother's womb.

Moving into such a beloved home has its challenges. To start, there is the guilt of locking my door in a community where doors are rarely locked, and knocking is something only outsiders do. Growing up, the little half-white girl in me once knocked so loudly on my best friend's door that her mom answered in a sheer panic. When she opened the door and saw me standing there, her face dropped and she scolded me "TAH! UNAPALUALUK PUKIQTALIUNASUGIQAUJAGIT!" Darn you! I thought you were the police! I thought you were a qallunaaq! Don't ever knock on our door again! We don't knock like that! Just take your shoes off and come inside." That was the only time she ever yelled at me. She was still amused and had a good laugh afterwards talking with my mother about my anxiety-inducing faux pas.

When I was a teenager, I never thought about others needing privacy. We grew up just walking into the homes of our friends and family, popping in or dropping by at our whim, having some tea, enjoying food, watching the programs on TV with each other, going on with life as though we were always expected to be a part of the day. Looking back, I think of how patient and kind my aunts, uncles, and older cousins were for letting me in and giving me a place to go. Whether or not they really offered it, the open door culture we've always lived in granted me a safe haven from the angst-ridden cabin fever of not having many hangout options besides my bedroom or my parents' living room.

As an adult, I can be intensely private and need the proper space to feel my feelings. I need room for my thoughts. I need to feel as though my space won't be invaded suddenly. This is not something that is promised here, this is the land of availability, not schedule. Being welcoming is a very, deeply ingrained Inuit value. Helping each other is how we survived for millennia. Although people might have been wary of strange, new people approaching a camp, they were still prepared with open arms in case it was a family who was hungry or in need. Inuit would not turn someone away as it could mean death. Things might not be as intense in modern times, but the act of being a warm, welcoming person is still highly respected.

My grandparents never locked their door. This house was the first place any of us visited as soon as we'd arrive in town, nearly the first house you see when you drive up the long gravel road from the airport. I felt sad for a long time when I considered that some people might drive by when they saw the house, knowing that my grandparents weren't there anymore. And other people might not come visit at all, for fear of falling into a heap of tears. While I understand so completely, it hasn't made the burden of their legacy any lighter. There are days when you think to yourself, I wish they were here instead of me and then other days where you are grateful for the peace of an uninterrupted day.

My grandparents always seemed to miraculously have enough love to feed any hungry soul. I know I fall short in many ways. How could I not? This house was the congregation place for not only their children, their children's children and beyond, it was a place anyone could come and eat, converse, sleep, find warmth and comfort. I struggle with simply doing the things I need to do to keep myself and my family happy, let alone an entire community of people. I can be so glaringly white in the way I present myself — finding the balance feels impossible when being qallunaaq is more than a skin colour — it's a state of mind and a way of being that is totally opposite of being Inuk.

There are days that it's nearly impossible not to think of them. They are in everything. I kneel by the bathtub to scrub the thickened rings. Preparing myself for a soothing bath, I suddenly find myself weeping. Struck by the simple thought of the remnants of their washing, of going through the monotony of their lives. The daily rituals of hygiene that fill up the hours, the things that make us human. The brushing of our hair, the washing of our bodies. I am overcome with visions of my grandmother in her last days, unable to care for herself.

I wish I had come home sooner. It's as though I am washing them away, washing away the last of their physical presence. How long will it be until I can no longer smell them?

It's strange the things that stay with you, like the thickened rings around the tub, the substance that holds fast against everything that would wash it away. Some memories are seared into your memory like a cattle brand. Some just flutter away like wisps of arctic cotton.

My grandmother's beauty secret, she told me as she leaned in close with a twinkle in her eye, was cocoa butter cream. She gently opened the container and smiled knowingly as though she held the secret to ageless beauty in her hands. She offered me some and we coated our faces in hopeful silence. Her skin always seemed so soft and glowing, the life force of her constant prayers humming underneath, like a thousand conversations with God vibrating from her pores.

In high school, a schoolmate had just returned from another community where she had attended meetings on the subject of healing. She had spoken to a woman who had told her that after you cry it's important to replace the water. I remember her saying passionately, that after a long cry you should go drink a glass of water, or take a shower, or wash your face to replenish your water and it will make you feel better.

> Some memories are seared in your memory like a cattle brand. Some just flutter away like wisps of arctic cotton.

As I sit kneeling by their tub, the last of the soapy film scrubbed away and slipping softly down the drain, I sigh heavily and wonder about the simple act of caring when actions speak louder than ambiguous feelings. There are times when my mind feels like a battering ram. Do we learn to care for ourselves by caring for others? How many times had I washed their tub before I lived here? Had I ever? How many times did I take the time to do the little things they needed done? To help them care for themselves? I had never really thought about it. I hadn't thought about the rings around their tub until it was mine. These thoughts make me yearn for another chance to wash their bath while it was still theirs. Another chance to sweep their floor and pour them a cup of tea. I get up and take a deep breath, not wanting to be consumed by remorse. I instead focus on what I remember, of what I have been given. The wisdom and strength imparted. It is the solid foundation of their lives that beats steadily in my heart, the memories that remind me of how simple acts of service are sometimes the loudest declarations of love. I pour myself a glass of water. I replenish loss with refreshment.

How simple it is to care for ourselves and yet we often forget the way. The white noise of expectations deafening the voice of our most instinctual knowledge.

As the days go on our own memories begin to sweep over the house like fresh coats of paint. We have a beautiful, vibrant baby boy who fills the house with his energy and enthusiasm. I never knew a love could exist that both terrifies and emboldens you. He makes every moment more meaningful and more challenging. Whether I soar or stumble, little eyes are watching and so instead I work at showing him a steady example. Steady with love, steady with emotion. He learns so quickly and amazes me with the depth of his grasp for anything I try and teach him. Mostly I want him to know how much I love him.

This house is now where he took his first steps, said his first words, fills the air with his shouts, squeals, cries, and laughter. The delicate threads of our lives are being woven together like a tapestry. The vitality of his life and our love for him is like a warm cleansing water washing over this house with newness.

One of the most surprising things of motherhood for me has been, there is no time for self-loathing. No time for the usual ruminations. Everything has to be more calculated, more timed. I thought it would mean less of me, and it has, but it's meant less of the stuff that doesn't matter. When I fretted that I might no longer be able to indulge in my every creative whim, Aaron gently reminded me, "If it's important to you, you will find the time for it." Words of wisdom are like water to the soul.

My thoughts always gently lean into them. I hear their voices, their stories... images of their bodies flash before me. One night in my sleep I can hear the sound of my grandfather's kamik clad feet sliding across the speckled vinyl tiles, a rhythmic swish, swish, swish as he walks to the kitchen to pour himself a cup of tea. Followed by the tink, tink, tink of his spoon against the cup as he stirs in spoonfuls of sugar. I sit up in bed, eyes wide open. Had I really heard him or was I dreaming?

I leave a light on and as I walk to another room, it's the middle of the night and I am alone in my wakefulness, but in the back of my mind I can see my grandfather pointing to the light, telling me to go back and shut it off. He was cautious with his electricity, a good caretaker over his household and he never tolerated lights left on carelessly. Be a good steward over the little things and you will become ruler over much. It's as though he speaks to me with every light I leave on and I turn back to switch it off because of him. These walls are talking again.

I stand in the kitchen with a glass of water in the near darkness. How many times I have longed to show my ataatatsiaq and my anaanatsiaq the things that I create, to introduce them to my son and to Aaron, to know that they would approve of me here in this space. A gradual but steady wave of relief rolls over me as I realize how much of them still lives on in me. How living here has allowed me to slowly forgive myself for not seeing the treasure that was right in front of me all along. To accept myself for who I am without comparisons to anyone, not even them. I think of the parts of them that are still very much alive, the memories linger like a sweet smelling incense. The smoke hanging in the air, suspended long after the embers have gone out.

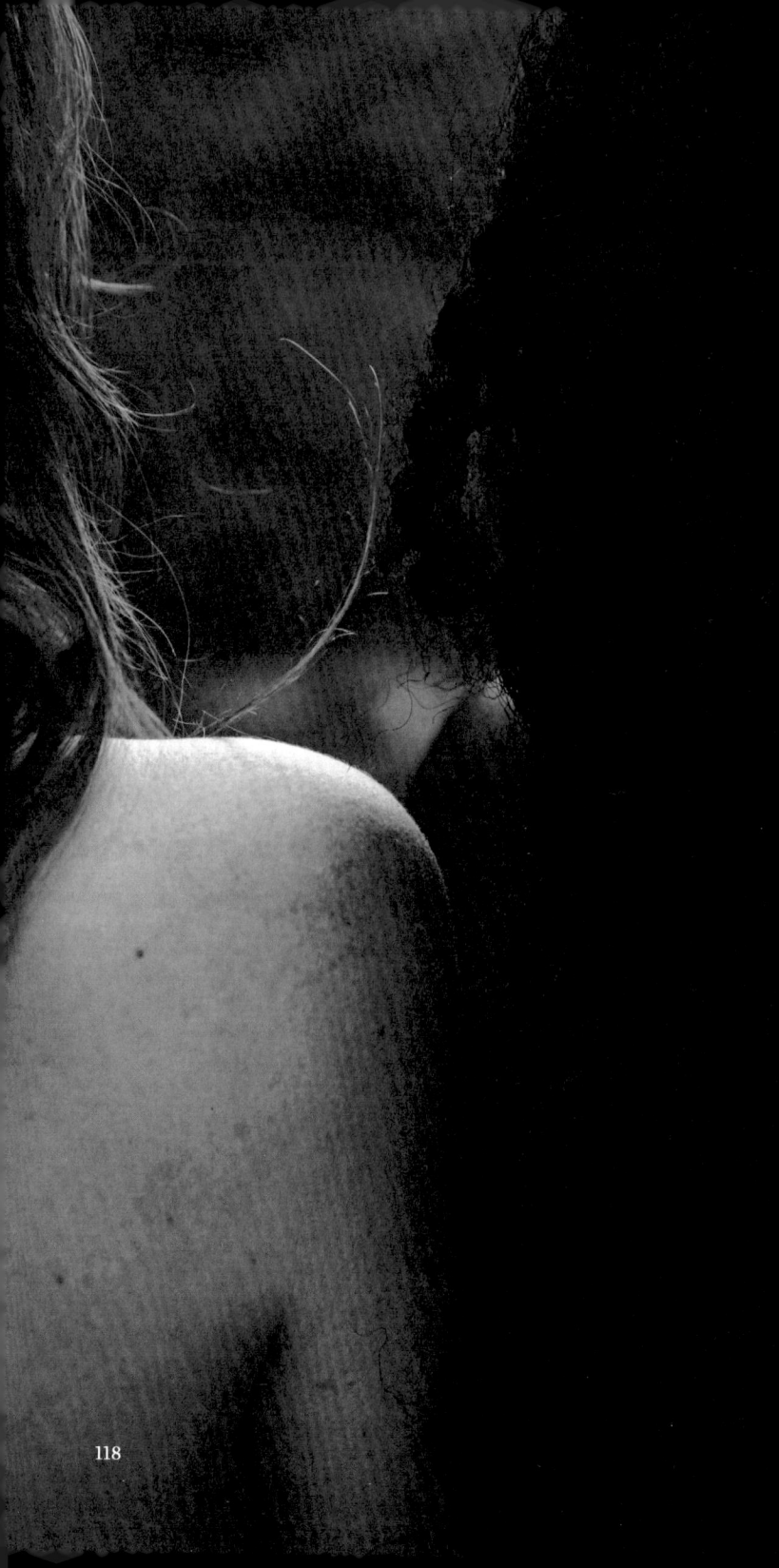

MO HANDAHU

will speak to you as if she's known you for several lifetimes—even if you've just met her. Mo immigrated to Halifax, Nova Scotia from Zimbabwe in 2005 and still calls the maritime province home. Her blog Lion Hunter celebrates eclectic style and she's written about style and plus-sized fashion for *People Magazine, Buzzfeed, Flare* and more. When I asked her to write a piece for this anthology she was hesitant at first. Mo was in the midst of processing an extremely traumatic experience—the loss of her yoga teacher, a close friend, when she was murdered in Spring 2016. Ultimately, Mo decided that the act of writing and submitting this short, lyrical piece of prose would be the first step towards coming to terms with her grief. A true act of self care.

The Place We Met
by Mo Handahu

I could barely walk by the place where we first met without feeling like my knees would buckle.

My heart forgot the rhythm of its beat, my eyes watered. Moisture covered my palms. The place we met — with its bright orange walls and the welcoming hug, our favourite heated room where we laid down our mats, where we were vulnerable but safe: Not our best, but getting better. This was a place that we shared with many, the place I held dearly as our place, but it now scared me. It scared me because I wasn't able to wrap my head around the painful truth that you wouldn't be here. That I wouldn't see your face light up, the way it used to, the very moment you saw me.

I allowed fear to take control of my heart, to inhabit me and take control of my emotions. I avoided our place. I took the longer route home. I needed to ignore the feeling of seeing your face everywhere, to overlook seeing the consistent kindness in the eyes of strangers, kindness that looked just like yours.

I wallowed and wallowed hard. Fear thrived and passion disappeared.

I knew I had to live, I had to find a way to thrive without fear. To flourish, to exist again, I knew I had to meet you, though you wouldn't come, to our place. I had to bravely look at our place, take in the brick and the murals, take in the smells and sounds until they were so deep in my soul, until my knees didn't buckle, until my heart caught up to its beat and until my eyes smiled again.

I took care of myself by moving forward and looking up, by acknowledging that I see you everywhere I go, by absorbing that genuine kindness I used to see in your eyes but now find in strangers along my path. I hope that anyone else who lost you and misses you, catches glimpses of you like I do, living within the things and people you left behind.

I am still meeting you at our place. I glance at the bricks and the mural with gratitude. I have a lot more peace in my heart. I keep looking to see you in others. I am meeting you, in my own way. ◗

Contributors

NADA ALIC
nadaalic.com

KATHRYN BONDY
@creweler

ADINA TARRALIK DUFFY
@adinaapplebum

TALLULAH FONTAINE
tallulahfontaine.com

MO HANDAHU
lion-hunter.com

JESSIKA HEPBURN
ohmyhandmade.com

LEAH HORLICK
leahhorlick.com

VICKY LAM
vickylam.com

ANGELA LEWIS
angelalewis.com

BROOKE MANNING
loommusic.bandcamp.com

SOFIA MOSTAGHIMI
sofiamostaghimi.com

NAOMI MOYER
naomimichelle.com

ANABELA PIERSOL
fieldguided.com

WINNIE TRUONG
winnietruong.com

CHRISTINA YAN
cargocollective.com/christina_yan

You Care *Too* Much

ERIN KLASSEN
editor
withoutpretend.com

JEN SPINNER
art director
jenspinner.com

LIRON DAVIS
publicist
@lironoffthecob

KAIT SOUCH
layout & design
kaitsouch.com

JULIA DE LAURENTIIS JOHNSTON
production coordinator
@juliadelj

Copyright © 2016 With/out Pretend publishing.
All rights reserved. Produced in Toronto, Ontario.
Printed by C.J. Graphics Inc.
Visit withoutpretend.com for more titles.

ACKNOWLEDGEMENTS

This book was possible because of many beautiful souls who are not formally credited on the contributors' page. Big thanks especially to Jill Wood and family, Brian Dort, Tanya Santos, Mary Shaw, Hazel Eckert, Laurie McGregor, Jim Kim and Joe Veroni.

Thank you for the beauty and bravery of our (anonymous) models for the photo series used throughout the book, *It's Only Natural*. Special thanks to Angela Lewis for photographing this series so beautifully. It was a joy to collaborate!

Thank you to our loving, patient and supportive friends and family who encourage us to make things and allow us to be wholly ourselves.

And, a final swell of gratitude for the remarkable, courageous women who contributed to this collection. Thank you for digging deep, taking risks, and trusting us with your stories. This book is published with the hope that others will benefit from the lessons you've learned and shared within these pages about what self care means, to you.